THE OTHER SIDE

A memoir of hope in the midst of depression

Acknowledgments

First I have to thank my Aunt Eileen, Uncle Padraic, cousins Sandra, Emma and David for giving permission to name their son and brother, my youngest cousin Noel. Their kindness opened up a world of memories for me, not least of me (as a child) visiting them in Dublin, and being introduced to their room-filling Lego city which they had housed in their attic – as a child, many hours were lost in wonder, enjoyment and imagination. They have also allowed me to keep Noel's beautiful memory alive, helping me convey an important message for you, the reader, and for this I am very grateful.

I am also very grateful to two fine professionals for generously giving me their time and expertise: Dr. Richard Blennerhassett and Dr. Claudia Marinetti.

I would also like to thank my excellent designers: Al Kennington (logo design) and Steve Langan (cover photographs).

Special thanks to the JM Agency, Publishing Consultancy team. Including Susan Lewando, Amanda J Evans and Joseph Youorski for their expert editing and advice, Parvathi N Venkitaraman for her professional cover, and to Jeremy for steering the ship so expertly — they make it all possible.

THE OTHER SIDE

*A memoir of hope
in the midst of depression*

Neil Kelders

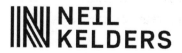

The Other Side

Published 2022 by Neil Kelders
Copyright © Neil Kelders

ISBN: 978-1-7391296-3-7

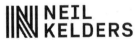

Disclaimer

The information in this book has been compiled by way of the personal experiences of the author, Neil Kelders, in relation to the specific subjects addressed, but is not a substitute and not to be relied on for medical, healthcare, pharmaceutical or other professional advice on specific circumstances and in specific locations.

Please consult your physician to ensure advice and tips given in this book are appropriate for your individual circumstances. If you have any health issues or pre-existing conditions, please consult your physician before implementing any of the information provided. This product is for informational purposes only and the author does not accept any responsibility for any liabilities or damages, real or perceived, resulting from the use of this information.

Some of the following description is raw and might be triggering, so read to the end, and don't take this as permission to act.

This work depicts actual events in the life of the author as truthfully as recollection permits. While all persons within are actual individuals, (some) names and identifying characteristics have been changed to respect their privacy.

Dedication

This book is dedicated to my mom, Breda Kelders with love. You gave us everything; we never wanted for anything. I don't know how you did it! This book is my way of showing you that I am now doing okay and that there is no need to worry about me. But as we all know mothers will always worry. I am living life my way, whilst being able to navigate whatever life throws at me. I got this. Thanks Mom, I love you.

In memory of my cousin Noel Daly.

Your Free Gift

As a way of saying thanks for your purchase, I'm offering this Neil's Notes Guided Exercises eBook for FREE to my readers.

To get instant access just scan this QR code:

 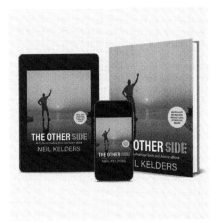

Inside the eBook, you will discover:

- All of the Neil's Notes which are dotted throughout this book
- How to develop these Neil's Notes and use them as tools in your daily life
- How to get started on your journey of self-help TODAY!
- And so much more

If you want to make the most of the advice and guidance in this book, make sure to grab the free eBook.

Foreword

Depression and anxiety are the most common expressions of mental suffering, of mental ill health in our world today. The World Health Organisation (WHO), which studies the impact of diseases, now ranks depression as the commonest form of disability worldwide, ahead of conditions such as cancer and heart disease. Depression and anxiety commonly occur together. In psychiatry it is unusual to see pure depression or pure anxiety. While a person may be designated as suffering from a depressive or anxiety disorder the person experiencing these conditions will usually experience a mix of symptoms of both. The pain and despair experienced by the sufferer may result in them ending their life through suicide.

The prevalence of depression and anxiety has increased worldwide in recent decades, particularly in the 21st Century. Ireland has not been spared. The crisis in our mental health services is ever in the background. On the personal level there is surely no family in Ireland that has not been touched by suicide, either through losing a family member, friend or someone they have known. Our common reaction to suicide is one of shock and disbelief, magnified when it appears in so many cases, that there were no signs of the underlying despair and suffering of the person before this fatal act, that to outer appearances all may seemed to have been going well in the person's life.

We live in an era where there is an increased awareness of the importance of mental health. People who have experienced mental ill health have shared their experiences, have written and spoken about their ordeal, treatment and eventual recovery. There are now many memoirs of depression. In approaching Neil Kelder's The Other Side, you may ask do we need another memoir of depression? The answer is a resounding YES. Neil has written a moving, funny, and at times painfully frank account of his experience of depression and anxiety. It is the finest account I have read of the state of mind that leads a person to see suicide as the only solution to their despair. Thankfully for Neil, he was able, with the support of a loving family, to step back from this irreversible step and start his slow journey to recovery and finding a life worth living. His account provides, not only an invaluable insight into the insidious nature of depression and anxiety, which are so often hidden, but, uniquely, it offers a practical guide to anyone struggling with depression or simply feeling stressed or experiencing feelings of not being good enough, to find joy and meaning in their lives.

In the introduction we are introduced to a young man on the eve of St. Patrick's day, sitting in his car after a normal day's work who writes, 'and instead of wondering what pub I will go to, I was deciding whether or not to end my life'. He tells us that this wasn't the first time in his life that he had wanted to die, but it was more real than ever before; that he has been struggling with such feelings from the age of 15 and now 21 years later he felt he was fighting a losing battle. He was physically and mentally exhausted from wearing a mask for years. You see Neil was a person who in public appeared outgoing, engaged in life and without a care in the world. The other side of the mask, his inner self, was a dark, fearful world where he struggled with feelings of anxiety, depression and suicidal thoughts, and a constant fear of being exposed as not being the confident person he presented to the world.

Neil's memoir relates an idyllic childhood in the Killarney of the late 1980's. He writes movingly of what, for a ten year old boy, was a soul destroying experience when his father left the family and how this affected him over his teenage years, sowing the seeds for the emergence of depression and anxiety. Neil's decision to reveal his inner turmoil, having come close at the age of 36 to ending his life, was a turning point in his battle against depression and anxiety, or, as he likes to term it, D&A. He started to record his experiences and this memoir provides a rich account of his search to find solutions and create a better life. His initial experience with an emphatic counsellor helped him understand his situation and that he was not alone. An important lesson from his experience is that it is important to seek professional help, but, alongside this, the person themselves needs to actively find ways to manage their own mental health, similar in the way to which we are encouraged to manage our physical health.

This manual provides a practical guide, not for defeating D&A, but in finding a way to live the life we wish while being able to manage the negative thoughts and feelings when they recur as they tend to do.

At the end of each chapter there is a section 'Neil's Notes', in which he invites the reader to consider how what he has shared might be relevant to their life and tips to change the situation. Another important message of the book is that one can change one's current situation and have a much better life, but as Neil says 'you need to take action'. This book shows how to do this.

Neil's memoir charts one man's journey from suicidal depression to living a rich and full life. He has moved from Ireland to living internationally as a successful personal trainer and life coach during the past decade.

Who should read this book? I hope it will find a wide audience among anyone struggling with depression, anxiety or stress, alongside those working in the field of mental health and education.

Neil himself believes we could all take something from it as mental health is part of our make up. I fully agree and Neil, as a personal trainer and life coach, has helped me to transform my life for the better over several years. He is a truly inspiring person and his book is a triumph of the human spirit.

Dr. Richard Blennerhassett MB FRCPsych FRCPI
Consultant Psychiatrist

Contents

PART ONE

The Beginning

Introduction
Time to close my eyes to the world

My feelings now: I'm ready to go. I do not want to be here anymore. I'm relaxed with that decision; I don't worry about dying. I just want to go. I'm tired and I just want to close my eyes to the world.

On the eve of St. Patrick's Day, or Paddy's Day as we Irish call our favourite national holiday, I came very close to ending my life. Paddy's Day is a time to celebrate our proud Irish identity, with family and friends. As night falls over Ireland and the wider world, people are having one or two pre-celebratory pints. By 10pm, most are in fine fettle and the towns and cities are buzzing. But as the world was lighting up, I was sitting alone in my car, outside my house. It was the end of a long day working with clients, and instead of wondering which pub I would go to, I was deciding whether or not to end my life.

Can you imagine feeling like this? Have you ever felt like this? Wait, are you feeling like this now? Do you know what I'm talking about? No? If not you, then maybe someone you know is feeling like this. No matter who it is, one thing we will all agree upon is that it's the most horrible of feelings; one which seems to be constant, with no end in sight. It's exhausting. All we want is for it to stop. We come to believe there is only one way out of this life sentence: The release of death.

It makes me sad to recall that I felt death was my only option, then, and to realise today that there are many people out there, now, thinking the same thing.

In this book, I will prove to you that there are other ways to cope with depression and anxiety. Even with all the pain and suffering you're going through, there is hope out there, all you have to do is step towards it. That said, I am not here to give people false hope. I am not here to end your depression and anxiety. I am here to show you how to deal with it, manage it, maybe give you that little bit of real, meaningful hope that can help you through it. I will bring you into my world and take you, step by step, through my journey with depression, anxiety, suicidal ideation, towards a better life. I will show you that there are ways or courses of action to deal with these struggles. Some of these actions will be with the help of others and some, believe it or not, are already within you. You deserve to explore these new courses of action, as do your family and friends, and they deserve to get the chance to help you. Can you imagine what it would be like for your family if they never found out about your pain until it was too late for them to help you?

This wasn't the first time in my life I had wanted to die, but it was more real than ever before. On that day I was at the end. I couldn't go on, and this continuous cycle had been slowly ripping me apart piece by piece, day after day since I was fifteen years of age. I sat in my car, mentally and physically exhausted. I wasn't able to 'do this anymore', to hide my true feelings, mask what is inside me, deal with the fear of being exposed. To my mind back then, there was no other way out of this, other than suicide. I had exhausted all the other options. Nothing worked. So, I took out my phone and hit record. For the first time I started to document my chronic battle with mental health problems.

I bet you're thinking: Neil, can I stop you there, please? What is the point in recording something that nobody would hear or see? You're right, I didn't record a message as a cry for help, I didn't want help; to be sure, I was beyond help. At that time, I was certain that *nothing* could be done for me. I was a lost cause. So why did I record it? In my mind I believed it would provide some comfort and answers to the people I would leave behind. The message was intended to explain to my family (my mother, brothers, sister-in-law, nieces and nephews), why I had to leave this life. I had tried everything, but nothing had worked. I wanted them to understand that I was exhausted, that the 21 years of fighting and battling this darkness had left me depleted and longing for peace. I couldn't do it anymore. Please, just let me die. Please. It's all I want.

Welcome to my world!

Neil's Notes

As you read through this book, you'll frequently come across the term 'mask' or 'masking'. I was always very careful to put on a fake front which allowed me to hide my true face, reflecting suffering. I would, in public, seem outgoing, funny, active, involved, not having a care in the world; forever seen as someone who was enjoying life. This could not have been further from the truth. This mask was donned every time I stepped outside my door; when meeting family, friends, work or at sports. I still wear it on those occasions when I just don't want people to see how I'm truly feeling. This is how I hid my struggles for over 21 years.

Are you wearing a mask? Do you call it a mask? If not, how do you describe it? Can you write down situations in your life when you put on your mask? Can you write down why you put it on in each of those situations? Do you know why?

—◆—

Chapter 1

Hi, I'm Neil Kelders. Sorry if I caught you off guard with my introduction, but isn't that what depression, anxiety, stress, whichever mental health problem you might be battling, or even life, does?

It catches us off guard.

You might be feeling, right now, similar to how I felt back in 2014 and the 21 preceding years. Whatever your reason, I'm glad that you're here, reading this book. Thank you. I mean it. THANK YOU; because by you being here and reading this book, I get another chance to talk and be heard. Even to this day, I sometimes forget to be open about my problems. As you turn each page, I'm being open with you, which in turn brings me great relief. Thank you!

I want to share with you my world of depression, anxiety, stress, and suicidal ideation; a 21-year journey that I tried to deal with alone, always in fear that someone would find out. I will try as best I can to explain the feelings each of my mental problems brought, and how I tried and failed to deal with them. Then I will take a look at the turning point in my life; the one which allowed me to sit here and write these words you're now reading. This is something I would once have believed was well beyond me. I believe this book can provide the hope you, or someone you love, needs, in order to face those demons and begin to feel worthy to live the life you or they want.

I would like to think that this book is for everyone, definitely for those suffering as I did, but also for those of you who are interested in gaining a deeper insight into the life of someone with depression, anxiety, and suicidal ideation, and learn how they cope, or, more often than not, don't cope, with this seemingly never-ending battle. Right now, someone, somewhere, is struggling badly; someone is contemplating suicide.

For years I fought a losing battle, 21 years to be exact. The first time I really became aware that there was something going on with me was when I was 15 years of age. I remember it as if it were yesterday. I was sitting at my desk in my bedroom at home in Killarney, Co Kerry. I was supposed to be studying (boy, I hated studying), but was in fact doing everything but. I was a great one for the preparation phase of study; getting everything organised, which, of course, could take a while, right? Obviously, when that was done, sure, didn't I need a break?

That particular evening, when I was eventually ready to start studying, I opened a book – a big, hefty science book, which I was unsuccessfully trying to revise. As per usual my mind began to wander and I started being creative with pencils, pens, markers, anything within reach really, scribbling down important details like the latest Liverpool Football Club best XI team, which I believed would win the English Premier League title that 1993/94 season (in hindsight not such a good prediction eh! They wouldn't win the title until the 2019/20 season).

I remember writing the word '*suicide*' in a very artistic design, followed by the words, '*to die*'. This wasn't a random, meaningless word to me; it had depth. It was a thought I had been having every day, many times a day. As a teenager, I had explored this thought of suicide so much that it had become very normal for me. In fact, I thought about it so much that I presumed everyone did. It wasn't until 21 years later, at a counselling session at Pieta House (Pieta provide counselling to those with suicidal ideation, engaging in self-harm, or bereaved by suicide), when my counsellor said, 'No, Neil, no, not everyone thinks about suicide.' That realisation really came as a surprise to me. And here was me thinking that at 36 years of age I had some ounce of intelligence, eh!

By the way, I think of my experience with depression and anxiety and suicidal ideation as a battle. Some might not, and some don't accept the use of this description, but I say 'tough' to those people. They were not in my mind and body, day after day, week after week, and year after year while I was trying to survive. It was very much a battle for me. Oh yeah and it's my book, after all, eh, so!

Being able to look back, somewhat objectively, I believe that my mental health problems started, or were at least triggered, much earlier than aged 15 years. Most likely by certain childhood traumas which were not dealt with. For years, I did not want to believe that those traumas or a certain person's actions could affect me so much, but I also wanted to believe that I was stronger than some 'minor' events in my childhood. I did not want to believe I could be so weak.

I still have a reluctance to tell people about my childhood traumas. They are nothing unique or shocking, in fact they are happening to thousands of families around the world every week. If I were to tell you about my triggers; stimuli (which can be a person, place, situation, or thing) that contribute to an unwanted emotional or behavioural response, you would probably shout, 'Cop on and grow up, you idiot!' Well, if you did, then that's exactly the fear of judgement which was, and still is, a barrier, for me and so many other people, to sharing our mental health problems.

My Dad left us.

There's nothing shocking or unique about that, right? But for me as a 10-year-old boy, it was soul destroying. It took me years to figure out that it was him rejecting me that led to me developing a fear of rejection that stayed with me for years. Thrown into the mix are, of course, environmental factors.

I grew up in Killarney, in Co. Kerry, a small town in Ireland, in the

1980's. Back then it was unusual for a husband to leave his wife and kids. In fact, I think we were one of the first families in my town to go through something like this. Even before he left us, we were the talk of the town. There were whispers behind our backs, rumours circulating about him and about our family. Locals knew about what was going on before any of us did. He cheated on my mother, and cheated us kids by leaving us alone to face the knowing eyes and the town gossips. You see, our surname is Kelders, which is not an Irish surname, and not common, so is easily identifiable, and in a small town – well you get the picture.

As long as I can remember, my father worked away from home. Places like Saudi Arabia, Morocco, London and Amsterdam. As a child I would get excited when he came back to visit. I got to show him all the things he was missing out on, and we tried to play father and son catch-up in the very limited time available. I would get him to drive me to training, to come watch my games, or take me to watch a game or to even just walk with him in town made me happy. I felt ten foot tall. Then, even those moments were taken away from me.

Leaving aside the trauma of dealing with my father, there were many moments created in my childhood which are beautiful memories I carry with me today. I was lucky enough to grow up in Killarney – if you haven't visited, you should. It's situated in the South West of Ireland, not too far from the sea, and is surrounded by beautiful lakes, rivers and mountains. It's home to Ireland's highest mountain, Carrauntoohil. It truly is an outdoor Mecca.

We lived in a cul-de-sac (yes very posh, eh?) of ten houses which were only a fifteen-minute walk from Killarney town. It was a new estate back when I was born in 1978, with young families filling the houses, ensuring that I had plenty of friends.

We lived in each other's pockets. On a Friday night we could be found hanging out at number 1, playing Nintendo, and listening to music. At number 2, we had access to new ideas brought from stateside by our new American neighbour; recording videos with an old clunky VHS camera or building a skateboard ramp. Each of the other houses, numbers 4 to 10 had kids of a similar age, bringing various skills to our 'gang'. We had the father at number 10 who had this amazing self-built workshop at the back of their house, which was the production line for many a weird but wonderful invention we dreamed up; and that was our crew.

Our location was prime for us kids, close to town yet, surprisingly, it was surrounded by farmers' fields and our very own Pig's Hill, christened so as it was a hill with a barn which housed pigs. Our adventures and devilment filled our days with endless hours of fun. We would leave home for hours on end and only arrive back when hungry, injured or on hearing the dreaded call echoing from our mother's voice rebounding through forests and fields as she stood at the front door of the house, "Neil, home time! Neil? Neil!" The worst sound ever!

I have so many beautiful memories of my childhood, which I carry with me even today. These memories are not only of my neighbourhood, but also of school, not the dreaded schoolwork of course, memories of playing sports, going to local discos and the customary hanging out in the town on a Saturday, hail, rain or snow! I had a regular upbringing filled with many happy times and beautiful friendships, immersed in a loving and supportive family.

Neil's Notes

You time! Humour me! Close your eyes and let your mind wander to some happy childhood memories, ah go on! You know, sometimes we forget those moments which gave us so much happiness. As adults we tend to leave those memories behind, which is quite sad. I have learned to tap into them and actually use them to bring me out of a low period. Try it the next time you feel a little down! Did you try it? What memory came to mind? Did it make you smile?

Chapter 2
Taking a stranglehold

People often find it difficult to understand what it's like to experience depression and anxiety. In turn, this lack of understanding by others is a fear that blocks us from opening up. As we're human, our experiences in this life, and what triggers our depression or anxiety, will differ to some degree. But I do think that we have some common experiences and traits which we can associate with our mental health problems. You might explain or interpret them differently than I do, but I believe my interpretation will resonate with you, and vice versa.

Depression and anxiety are not just stand-alone conditions, they come with a lot of baggage which adds to and prolongs the suffering. Many of us will experience both depression and anxiety. On a given day our anxiety can be triggered and just when we feel we are coming to the end of the struggle, the depression consumes us. This, I find, can also happen in the reverse.

It usually happens to me when I've a bad night's sleep. I will start off anxious in the morning, try to manage it, but the anxiety pushes me towards a depressive state. The anxiety is brought on by fatigue, and the worry of not being productive the next day, which leads to a deflated and defeated feeling, ensuring my day is lost. I could not seem to break from this constant cycle of depression.

My darkness

Christmas Day 1984 was just around the corner; I was six years of age, and full of excitement. I loved Christmas Day. I would wake up early, usually around the 3am mark, and race into our sitting room, over to the tree and plug in the lights to reveal our stockings. Yeah, each of us had a big plastic stocking filled with gifts. Before digging into my stocking, I would race to the sitting room windows which looked out into our street, and from there I could see the lights of the other houses, indicating whether my friends were up, or not. If not, then that meant I was the first to wake on Christmas morning. I'm not sure if this was a known challenge amongst us, or just one I set for myself, but I'll tell you I was kicking arse year-in, year-out!

Our parents were great for presents. We would have our main present, the one we asked Santa for and maybe a surprise, or a Beano, Dandy or Liverpool FC Annual. This would be topped up with stocking fillers; little nick-nacks such as a colouring set or a small toy car. Oh, the excitement! I was lucky to have Killian and Paul as brothers, five and ten years older respectively, because their presents were always top notch. Killian always came up with the best ideas, you know that person who gets you something you didn't even know you wanted. Paul always came up trumps with a Liverpool jersey. Heaven!

In the lead up to this particular Christmas my parents sat myself and my two brothers down to tell us we were going to spend Christmas in Galway City and stay in the Great Southern Hotel in the city centre. This was so exciting. Nobody I knew ever did something like this, especially in the '80's. As I sat with this excitement, it quickly became an uneasy feeling. I didn't know anyone in Galway. I would be away from my friends, as we always hung out and marvelled over each other's presents.

Then it dawned on me, 'No, we can't go,' I said. 'Santa won't find us.'
My parents took me aside and reassured me that they had attached

a note to my letter to Santa, explaining all, and adding in the Galway address. After some coaxing or, as my parents would say, some reassuring, I was on board, and once again excited about our Christmas adventure.

So, I set about gathering up all the essentials. As a young fella 'essentials' meant clothes, teddy, of course my football, and pillow and duvet for the long trip ahead. As the youngest, I was stuck in the middle seat (such a crap seat, eh?), with my two brothers sitting like gods next to the windows, dictating when we shall have air and when we shall have warmth. Thank the heavens for my pillow and duvet! This was the time before motorways, so we drove along good ol' Irish roads and arrived in Galway City around five hours later.

Our car journeys were always made a little easier by my mother's treats. Every long trip we would take as kids, be it to my grandparents' house in Tullamore, Co. Offaly, or to visit my brothers in boarding school, or this trip to Galway, she would have some sandwiches prepared with some dessert, which could be anything from chocolate brownies, to scones to even a full apple tart and whipped cream. My mouth is watering with the very thought of those treats!

The excitement was building as we neared Galway City with the thought of Christmas Day fast-approaching coupled with the fact that we were going to spend it in a hotel! After some dinner we settled into our rooms, exhausted. I made sure to be in bed early so that I could wake bright and early for SANTA.

My eyes open, I'm still sleepy, and then it hits me: CHRISTMAS! SANTA! I hop out of bed and make my way to the Christmas tree. That has to be one of the best feelings I had as a kid. That Christmas I had asked the big man for a rally car, and there it was, under the tree in all its glory, my brand-new plastic rally car, pedals and all. I can still see its blue body, black steering wheel and black seat. It had this orange visor, to protect me from the elements of course. It was amazing! What made it even better, was that I had the best rally circuit a six-year-old boy could ask for: The hotel corridors, I mean WOW! I would race around terrorising (only kidding-ish) the poor guests, up and down the corridors, entering the elevator for 'repairs' and exiting as fast as my little legs could pedal, heading back out to the circuit (corridors) of another floor. Oh, the joy! After so many hours of pure hyperactivity, exhausted, I slowly drove my new but already worn car into its parking spot next to my bed. What a day I'd had! I lay in my bed with the biggest smile, an overtired but very happy little boy, closing my eyes, and dreaming of what tomorrow would bring.

'Mom'. I shout out as I lay in my bed.

'Mom?' There was no answer as I lay in the darkness with my eyes open. I sit up in the bed. 'Mooooooooom…' I waited patiently for five seconds. 'MOM!' Four seconds. 'MOM, MOM, MOM,' in a rhythmic tone, but there was no answer. Like what the heck? Where is she? Moms are supposed to come when called, aren't they? I sit alone in this big bed, in a dark unfamiliar room. I've had a bad dream. There's nobody coming to help me. I try to make sense of the room, tapping into my memory of the layout. Where is the door? The window?

Becoming more anxious, I can't figure out the room.

'Mooooooooom, Mooooooooom…'

I stop, listen, and again nothing. Now, even more anxious, my little heart thumping faster in my chest, I can feel the lump in my throat, you know the one you feel just before you're going to cry. One last go, 'Mooooooooom!'

NOTHING! Nobody hears me! I need someone! Nobody is there! I have a choice to make, stay where I'm and keep shouting out for my mom, or try something else. That something else was the decision to leap out of bed. A leap with a big enough spring so as to ensure that I have enough distance between myself and the bed, so that the monster underneath the bed can't grab my ankle as I try to make it to the safety of the door. I land on one foot and one knee, like an American Footballer getting ready for a play. The carpet softens the landing, and

I dash towards the door and slam into it on impact

'YES!' I made it, I'm safe, as I try to open the door. Wait, what? Where is the handle? I CAN'T FIND THE HANDLE!

Has this ever happened to you? You are half asleep as child, or as an adult, maybe after a few pints, and you can't find the handle of the door? You know it's there, but for love nor money you can't find it.

Now, let's take a step back for a second, and ask what was happening. I know the handle is there and I know it works, so why is it not working for me? Why, now, in my time of need, can I not find it? How is this possible?

This analogy is about life. There are going to be times when you try courses of action to help yourself but they don't seem to have the desired effect, so you think them useless to your struggle. Similarly, if you're looking for help with your struggles and feel you have been let down, not finding the right help, don't give up. You will find the help you need, just give it a little time and be consistent in your search.

Do not give up.

The help is out there for you, just as the handle really was on that door. I just had to take my time and find it.

I'm searching in complete darkness for the handle. Come on, where is it? My panic grows, I look behind me every so often to make sure no monster is sneaking up behind me. My search is futile, I can't find it. There is no handle. 'Mom,' I shout again, as I slap the door, which lead into the suite area of the apartment, in a last gasp of hope, 'Mom.'

Nobody comes. Nobody hears my cries. I'm alone.

I slump to the floor defeated. There are too many elements for me to battle; the darkness, the layout of the new room, no door handle and nobody hearing me. I can see light under the door; I know there are people out there. I can hear cars on the street, I can hear people passing in the corridor, but why can't you hear me? I know people are all around me.

Can't you hear me? Can't you see me standing here in the dark?

Lost, defeated, not knowing what to do, confused as to why you don't want to notice me, confused as to why you don't care about me, as to why you don't want to help me. I want to be helped, I do, I really do! Now, in tears, I believe there is no more I can do; I've tried everything, there is nothing more I can ever do to change this, it's my reality now; the darkness, the panic, the loneliness, the struggle.

This is my reality. This is what my mental health problems led me to believe. This is what I lived, alone, for over 21 years. The darkness, the pain, the constant battling to keep standing amongst you. As the world went on around me, I sat in my darkness, wanting to die.

Neil's Notes

Do you think I tried everything? Me, that six-year-old boy in that room, did I try everything? Yeah? No? If you say no, what more could I have done? Put down the book for a second or two and have a little think. Don't worry, I'll wait for you 😊

Did you come up with the same ideas as I did?

I could have stopped looking for that bloody door handle and looked for the light switch instead, and light would have ensured that I would find the handle of the door. I could have banged on the door to the corridor. I could have raced to the window, opened the curtains to let the light from the street brighten the room. There are so many things I could have done. They might not have solved all my problems but would have eased my panic and maybe led to someone reaching out and helping me or even finding my mom for me.

What more can you do, right now, to help yourself?

Again, put down the book, make a list, then take one of the points today and act on it!

—◆—

Reading this, you might understand that feeling of being trapped as the world continues on around you. You are quietly screaming for help, but it's falling on the deaf ears of your loving family and friends. This dark room is what is inside us. The failure to escape because we believe we're trapped by darkness, is real. All we can do is close our eyes and ride out the storm and hope for the best, knowing that it will all happen again and again and again.

Welcome to my world of over 21 years.

This is how best I feel I can explain my battle. It might resonate with you if you've walked or are walking in similar shoes. If not, then this hopefully highlights to you what I, and so many others, battle most days. The struggle is real, it's exhausting both mentally and physically.

Sorry, I just realised I left you hanging. My mom did come back to the room. So, what happened was, in the hotel there was a lady who'd look in on kids for the parents who were having dinner in the dining room, which was a very common thing to do back then. She sent for my mom, who immediately came to the room. I raced into her arms and got that mom-hug, where you feel so safe and can breathe again, knowing that everything will be ok. As I write this, I can still feel my head nestled into my mom as she kisses the top of my head. SAFE!

I know this might be hard to believe, when you're depressed or anxious and there seems like no end in sight, but there is always something we can do. When we are in the moment, it seems impossible, that there is no way out; but you have to believe me: There is a way to live with it, and there is that *someone* waiting to give you that mom-hug you so deserve.

Masking the truth

My go-to trick, which kept me 'safe' for most of my life, was the ability to hide my true self. Safe from what? If I'm honest – nothing; just my belief of a perceived judgement by you all, safe from a fear of admitting I'm different, safe from a fear of being looked on differently.

This is what I thought it meant, to keep myself safe, but the truth was, it only enhanced my problems, and distanced me from others. It delayed me from getting the help and support I needed. It stopped my life in its tracks. I wasn't really living at all, not pursuing relationships, not enjoying more moments with friends, not travelling to experience other cultures. I have labelled the time behind my mask as 'my lost years'.

Do not let this happen to you.

Step out from behind the mask.

I did a talk in a secondary school in Co. Cork, a few years back with transition year students (around 16 years old), to share my story and experiences, which was really engaging, surprisingly enough. After the talk the teacher, also my friend, Hughie, sent me a few words which I share on my social media platforms and website: How can the popular kid, the jock, the joker, the bright guy, the quarterback (actually wingback in Gaelic football), suffer from bad thoughts in his head? Surely, it's the kid with social, family, personal, academic, or alcohol or drug problems that gets these mind traumas?

Not so.

These words are from a friend, someone who has known me for many years. This is what he saw in me. This is what he remembers from meeting me every day when we were in school. This, for me, highlights just how hard I worked to ensure I never let my guard down, ensuring that nobody ever knew what was really going on behind the mask of the 'popular kid', the 'jock', the 'joker'.

Those school days were many moons ago, and that mask stayed

up for over 20 years. The energy and consistency to do that day in and day out for so long was exhausting. Surely it could not go on forever? Something had to give. And it did. I wanted an out, to be free from this life. I wanted to die, to end twenty years of pain and suffering. Strong words and strong thoughts, but that was my reality, then. Thankfully this want did not materialise and I'm still here to tell my tale. However, if I'm truly honest, now and again that mask makes an unwelcome appearance: Those times when I'm in a new setting with new people, and self-doubt kicks in; times when I'm asked to deliver a talk to a company, and thoughts of being exposed as an imposter rip me apart; times when I put off going deeper in a relationship because I believe nobody could love me. Luckily, today I can identify these moments and intervene and change my thinking behind them.

Reading this, you might say I wasn't very different from other kids growing up. I was active and seemingly connected to people and my environment, but sadly that wasn't so. I didn't really feel a connection to anything, and those kind words from Hughie, unbeknownst to him, best describe my skilful masking. A trait which I've used through the years, from my teenage, to college life right through to present day adulthood. I was, in fact, disconnected from life, even when I was being active or involved. Throughout my whole life, whether it was as a kid, a teenager, a student or an adult, I wanted to fit in, be 'normal', but I felt so disconnected at times from life, even when I was being active or involved. This reminds me of an acting workshop I was attending during which a friend of mine was taking photos of participants. He had snapped one of me while we were seated in a circle, listening to the facilitator explaining the format for the day. The photo captured my struggles that day perfectly. I had been looking forward to this workshop for a few weeks. I remember that day so clearly. It had been at least a year since I first revealed my mental health problems, and that week I was just living for this Saturday and the workshop. It could not come around quickly enough. When the Saturday finally arrived,

I woke up to a feeling of anxiety.

Has that ever happened to you? You wake and feel anxious or low, seemingly for no reason whatsoever.

You see, I would not only get anxious about uncertain future events, but I would also become anxious before well-planned events or activities, even the ones I was very excited to be attending.

I set about trying to calm myself. I made decisions which I felt would help me become more stable and at ease. I took the bus rather than driving to the course. While sitting on the bus on my way to town I could feel my anxiety building. It soon consumed my whole body. I was jittery; it was consuming me physically, a rapid heartbeat, sweating, the shakes, and internally with an explosion of negative thoughts. I wanted to exit the bus and skip the workshop I had been excited about for weeks.

I had to interrupt this anxiety, I had to take back some control over the situation. I called myself aside (an Irish way of saying I had to have a chat with myself) and tried to change my narrative. 'Neil, if you don't go, you'll become depressed and low, which will be a much worse experience.' I diverted my focus from myself to what was outside the window of the double-decker bus. There was a park, with a rugby game going on, people walking, brown leaves on a tree. Slowly, but surely, it was working. I was regaining some control. I hung on and arrived at the venue.

I walked in, still a little shaken and anxious from the bus ride, nodded politely before taking my seat and pretending to be busy on my phone, only so as to avoid eye contact and any possibility of anyone noticing what was going on behind my eyes. I knew most of the people at this course, but it didn't alleviate my feeling of anxiety, or release the dread hanging over me. I probably came across as a dick, when all I was doing was trying to fight the internal struggle, and give myself every chance of staying in the workshop for the day. So even with empty eyes and limited communication, that day was a win for me. My mind might not have been fully engaged, but I was there; present and accounted for. This was a win for me because as long as I could remember, I have, when in a similar state of mind, blocked myself from the world and ended up in bed, in darkness, waiting for my anxiety and depression to give me a reprieve.

If you've seen me in public, or been on a course with me or met me in some other situation and I seemed distant, impolite, then I'm sorry. I wasn't being rude; I was just using every last ounce of energy I had just to be physically present.

So, the next time you feel that someone is being an asshole, give them the benefit of the doubt. You never know the fight they have going on inside.

Neil's Notes

Take a look at the photograph of me in the workshop [refer to the Neil Note's Guided Exercises eBook P.13]. What do you see? Can you write down a few of the things you see from this photo? Look at my eyes, what story are my eyes telling? The eyes never lie, and assessing them can help us notice and become more aware of each other. The eyes reveal the struggles we hide. The next time you're talking to someone, look at them, take them in, stay present and really notice them. Start today!

—◆—

One small step for you
One giant step for me!

Have you met me? I'm apparently a very active, productive, outgoing, social, funny (if I do say so myself), empathetic, and an all-round cheeky messer. As my aunt Róisín (RIP) used to say to me, when I would joke and have fun with her, 'You are so bold!' (pronounced BAULD - an Irish term of endearment when being naughty).

As a kid, I remember being nicknamed Smiler by the uncle of a kid I knew from a rival football team. I've had people say to me that I inspired them as I was so productive, always doing something and thinking ahead. Telling me it's great to see that I'm so confident and progressive.

If only they had known, eh!

That explains why people were so shocked, and are still shocked, when I tell them that I suffer from depression, anxiety and suicidal ideation. People who have known me since I was a kid just couldn't comprehend what I went through.

I would like to tell you that this has all changed, and that it's me, Mr. Confident, writing this book. But as I sit here in a co-working space in Cyprus, six years after revealing that I have mental health problems, I still, at times, have to fake this confidence. Not always, mind you. I have become more confident for sure, but there are times when I falter.

It actually happened recently.

I made the decision in November 2020 to move to Cyprus, indefinitely. I didn't buy a return ticket. A big step for me, personally, but an action step that highlights my personal progress. I moved to Cyprus because Ireland was about to enter COVID-19 lockdown number two. I had successfully navigated my way through lockdown number one, with the aid of an online running challenge I was participating in with friends from Ireland and others from around the world. Between running and work I was kept busy and focused.

However, with lockdown number two drawing close, I knew this one would be a very different experience for me, for a number of reasons; it was heading into winter, with shorter days, and dark, colder nights. I was now injured, damaging the meniscus in my knee, and I could not run as before. I shared a house, so finding alone-time would be more difficult. I could feel my anxiety levels rising, way before the lockdown was imposed.

I knew I needed to make a decision, one which would push me outside my comfort zone. I decided to move to Cyprus, to create a better environment for myself during this lockdown. An important step for me, both for my mental health and my personal development. It was made possible for me to do my work online, ironically made possible thanks to COVID, so I took action and booked a one-way ticket to Cyprus.

I set off on my travels alone, which I didn't mind at all, because this time it was my decision to be alone. But I had made sure to set the goal of meeting new people and making new friends. This would be essential in order for me to remain in a positive mindset and find my feet in Cyprus.

Neil's Notes

I've constantly set myself challenges in order to build my confidence, strength and resilience. These challenges also allow me to learn more about myself and how I react in many different situations. It opens me up to a very different world. My challenge here was to meet new people. Can you pick a challenge for yourself? Maybe you text or call a friend you have not been in contact with for a while.

Start small. Try it today!

— ◆ —

With the goal of meeting new people in mind, I set about researching co-working spaces in Cyprus, and joined one in Paphos, which lies on the west coast. Co-working spaces are essentially shared workspaces. They offer office space or shared desk space for those looking to escape the isolation of a home office. These shared workspaces often have amenities such as coffee docks and organised social outings.

As you can tell I was trying to give myself every advantage in this 'people-meeting' challenge. In this space I would meet people from many different countries but with a similar mindset, plus they seemed to be very active with many group activities taking place amongst the members.

Week one, no friends made.

Week two, no change.

Week three, as the song goes, 'all by myself'.

Week four; pretty similar.

Four bloody weeks and nothing. What was going on eh? Well, I'll tell you what was going on. I was reluctant to go into the co-working space. Even though I had paid for the month, I had only been inside a handful of times, and those handful of times were in the evening when it was much quieter. I didn't want that feeling of all-eyes on me, I wanted to somehow just blend in without being noticed, which wasn't very conducive to making friends!

I was nervous, like being a kid on their first day in a new school. I did eventually gain in confidence (well less thinking and more doing), and began to use the space more and during times when it was busier. I began to chat to some people and was even invited to go to the roof-top on Friday as they have after work drinks there. Perfect, I thought, I'm up for that, this is it, a new me, meeting new people, possibly new friends. Wow! I've come a long way, I thought to myself. I was proud.

Friday arrives. It was 4pm and people had already gone to the roof for beers and a chat. I shut down the laptop and made my way to the stairwell. As I ascended the stairs to the roof, I could smell the barbeque going. As I climbed some more steps, I could hear the music, and as I neared the entrance to the roof, I could hear voices and laughter.

I stopped, more like, froze, for what felt like an age. Then I turned around and descended the stairs quickly, so that nobody would see me. At the time of writing, I was 42, and I still froze. It would take another two weeks before I worked up the courage to open the door to the roof and to more possibilities.

Pushing open that roof-door opened up a new Paphos to me, actually a new world. I had a Friday night outlet after a week of work. Somewhere to chat with many like-minded people. I was introduced to people from all over the globe; Germany, Denmark, Bosnia, Eastern Europe and China, Russia to Australia and New Zealand, to name but a few. I was even invited to Christmas dinner by virtual strangers – I couldn't believe it!

It might seem that the decision to leave Ireland for a few months during this world crisis was a no-brainer. For me it was still a tough decision to make. My fear of the unknown, the negative scenarios and outcomes that I would have myself believe, complimented with a splash of imposter syndrome (a belief I wasn't actually able to do these things), all dragged and poked their way into my decision-making process. It's amazing how I'm able to stand in my own way, blocking attempts to improve my well-being, and essentially my life.

I knew, when coming to Cyprus, that I would be going to a place where I knew nobody. I might easily stay within my shell, and not gain the confidence to put myself out there and meet people. I knew, even though the sun might shine, that my darkness could, once again, become more frequent and much darker. I knew I was leaving my safety net of family and friends, and I would have to discover some courage, and take more risks. This decision to go to Cyprus was very much a risk, but something I needed to do. I needed to move out of this unwanted comfort zone I had wrapped around me.

This new Paphos (since opening the door to the rooftop), has brought me hiking on trails throughout Cyprus, visiting local beaches for volleyball and other such activities, as well as simply enjoying a beer while watching the sun go down. Such an easy step for many can be a huge step for many more of us. But that one step has allowed me to grow. It has allowed me to find the confidence to stay longer in Cyprus, and even think of other places to visit. I've realised that I don't have to go back to Ireland. I can, if I want, move elsewhere; why not Bali or Malaysia? This one step has also made sure I haven't allowed myself to fall back into my dark hole. But I know I will face yet another internal conflict when it's time to make another decision. Such are the remnants of depression and anxiety.

Chapter 3
The grip tightens

Feeling worthless.

I'm a piece of shit. I don't belong breathing the same air as you. I'm worthless. This feeling is the worst of the worst, would you agree? When you believe this, then why try to help yourself? There is no point. The fact is you just don't belong, you don't fit in anywhere. Not at home, not at school, not at sports, no group whatsoever, not this world or this life.

I know people see this in me, they know I don't belong. They know I'm different; I'm odd, a person not worth getting to know. They are right, even though now and again I have a flicker of belief that I'm a good person. I'm someone you could like, I promise. But deep down I know they are right to pass me by.

I'm of the opinion people have no time for me, they don't give a fuck about me. They distance themselves from me. It goes without saying that it would not matter whether I lived or not. So then my beautiful mind goes into overdrive 'knowing' that people dislike me, and comes up with the solution: Why bother? Why bother trying to fit in, achieve things, it would be a futile exercise? Just give up and save yourself much heartache and pain. Maybe it's time to close my eyes to the world.

Holy crap, right? That escalated quickly. Welcome to my thoughts. A constant replay, day in, and day out, for over twenty years. But are these thoughts all in my head? Are they scenarios and judgments I assume or is there some foundation of truth to them? I definitely know my head runs away with itself, but I still buy into it. There have been certain incidents, where people made me feel so worthless, which have stayed with me over the years. One in particular comes to mind, it made me feel so inadequate and inferior. Man, I can still feel it now as I write these words. Soul destroying!

It was Christmas time, a few years back. It must have been, jeez, it must have been 2006 (many years ago and I'm still hanging onto it). We were in a late bar in Killarney town. Traditionally a night over the Christmas holidays, when all locals around my age would go to this certain bar, The Laurels, as a kind of annual reunion; meeting with old school friends and catching up on life. I had started chatting to a friend, Con, a lovely guy, and I was enjoying this meet and catch-up after so many years. He then introduced me to another old classmate, Pat, and proceeded to inform this other guy that I was studying law. We are standing near the bar, loud Christmas music ringing in our ears but I can feel my heart pounding my chest, nearly to the point that I can hear it beating, even with the music blaring.

I will never forget this guy's response. It was that look he gave me; you know the one, the '*you* doing law?' look, one of utter disbelief, followed by his actual words, '*You* doing law'. It cut me like a knife. I felt like a total and utter shit. I wanted to jump him and beat him, the arrogant prick. But all I could do was stand there in all of my worthlessness.

I felt that his reaction mirrored what all the others were thinking, that I was a waste of space and would never amount to anything. He judged me because of what he remembered from our school days. I had been a messer, not too studious and always up for the craic. He had been the total opposite. His judgment of me had never changed. I have never felt so small, so worthless. It was a very hard knock to take and one, well as you can tell has stayed with me.

Today, that incident doesn't have the same effect on me, but is a reminder to myself that I now don't give a shit what people think. Okay, maybe sometimes I do, but the important thing now is that I certainly don't allow it to affect me. I now know that what I want and think is far more important.

But you know what? Words do bloody matter and they matter a lot more depending on the relationship you have with the person who expresses them. Choose your words carefully. You never know who they might cut.

Beating myself up

Boy oh boy, was I hard on myself and, I must confess, still am at times. D&A (Depression and Anxiety) get such a stranglehold that it starts to affect every aspect of your life. You become frustrated and angry at the fact that you're a useless waste of oxygen. It got to the stage where I would question why I should bother doing anything. What was the point when I fuck everything up? Do you know what I mean?

That voice in your head, constantly nagging at you. Why bother getting out of bed? Why bother getting dressed? Why bother going outside? Why bother meeting people? Why bother with anything as you make no impact on anybody's day? Why bother it will just end in disaster? Why bother? Why bother? Why fucking bother?

But even when you do manage to take some sort of action to get yourself moving, and it seems that you might just be turning a corner, BANG! You fail. You are in a state of shock. You believe you did everything within your power to avoid failure, to avoid disappointment. You become overwhelmingly disappointed and angry when the expectations you've set yourself are not met. Once again, you've failed. You come down on yourself like a ton of bricks. Even if something outside of your control disrupted your path to succeeding. It doesn't matter, you lay the blame firmly at your doorstep.

On reflection, most of these situations were doomed from the outset. If I'm totally honest, I didn't put in the work or time required to succeed in the first place. So how the hell could I expect to succeed? I've done this so often. So many times, I set myself up for a fall. Self-sabotage.

Looking back on it, I was very angry in life, particularly with myself. I could see no good in my life, no good in me living. I felt such a waster, not achieving or making anything of myself. I seemed to be going around in circles. Everyday seemed like Groundhog Day. The same old routine. Nothing to wake up for in the morning. Nothing to stimulate me each day.

Life was passing me by. On the odd occasion, I would try and propel myself out this rut, but my half-arsed attempts were futile. I would inevitably fail, which I coined 'the story of my life'. Those failures hurt; each one left a mental scar. Failures led to frustration and was followed by anger leading to dark lows. A continuous cycle for many years.

I feel reluctant to write this. But even sitting down to write this book has not been plain sailing. I've stopped and started so many times. Writing a book is something I wanted to do for so long, but I kept blocking myself, telling myself that someone like me can't write a book. Who in the wide earthly world would want to read this trash? Who would even care about my story? So, Neil, do yourself a favour and quit this delusional dream.

Each and every day I have to overcome these thoughts and this internal struggle. They raise their ugly head not only before I sit down and begin to write but also throughout the writing process. It could be an hour into it, two hours or ten, it doesn't matter, they will come. I might have been progressing well with the writing but thoughts are always lurking: Failure, imposter, fake, delusional…

This was the story of my life. It's an exhausting struggle and one which for so many years got the better of me. But, I'm glad to say, if you're reading this book, then you now know I've won this particular struggle. Go me! The secret?

Take it one struggle at a time.

Expectations

My expectations for my life were grounded in what I believed I saw in other people's lives. Do you ever wish you could have someone else's life? I did, all the time. From what I could see, all those with whom I crossed paths, had it figured out and were living their best life. This heightened my feeling of inadequacy and instilled a belief that I wasn't 'normal' nor would I ever be. I constantly compared myself to others. Compared myself to what I observed from the outside, believing that what I saw on the outside must totally be reflected inside each and every person. Sure, after all, doesn't my exterior mirror what's going on inside? Oh, wait! No, it doesn't!

Have you ever been crazy enough to have a notion that you would love to be an actor, rock star or that high-flying businessman or woman, only to bring yourself back to your reality, because to even think such a thing for yourself is laughable? Success is for THEM, those people, not for someone like me or you, right?

Just as most of us believe that achieving such a success is out of reach for someone like us, I believed that any achievement at all was out of my reach. Everything from a job interview, to asking a girl out, to making a starting position for a sports team, were all unattainable. I would tell myself there was no point in even trying, because it was obvious the answer would be a resounding 'no'.

Well, let me tell you a little secret, the majority of people, be they famous or not, they were and *are* like you and me. They are regular people, finding their way through this life. The difference is that the actor you admire or the entrepreneur or A-student you're looking up to actually went for it. They found something they wanted and decided to go for it. Against all odds.

I used to be very jealous of such people (people in a better place than me) thinking 'Oh, they have the life, it's so easy for them.' I can assure you that for 99.9999% of them it wasn't, it was a struggle, is a struggle, but they kept moving forward against all the odds, because it's what they wanted for themselves.

So why can't I do this? Why can't you do this? We believe we can't. We struggle to just get through each day. Yes, I have dreams, visions of where I want to be. But getting knocked down and rejected so many times (mostly by myself) takes its toll. I can't deal with any more knocks or failures, so I stop. I stay in my little (so-called) comfort zone. Which I should be thankful for, right? Who am I to want something different to everyone else? Just follow the herd, Neil, even if it's detrimental to your health. If it's good enough for them, it's good enough for you.

I followed this mistaken belief for so long. Not living how I wanted to live, not really doing what I wanted to do. Just doing enough to get by, following what society seems to tell us to do: Get a job, pay the bills, buy a house and a car, get married, work on weekdays, live for Friday; have your nice two-week holiday in the summer, and you'll even get some time at Christmas for a break. Sure, what more would you want? Be grateful for what you have (yes, it's important to be grateful – unless it's NOT what you want!), and when you retire you can do what you want, when you want.

I truly believe this limiting of myself contributed to my depression and anxiety. It's NOT what I wanted, I always wanted something different for myself. I didn't want to be stuck in an office. I didn't want to buy a house in one place and let that be it. I didn't want to live for the weekends. I didn't want to just have two weeks of holidays a year. But I believed this was the way it was supposed to be, so I questioned myself. 'Hey, why can't you just be like everyone else and get on with it and be bloody happy?'

Am I wrong to want something different for myself?

Do you get what I'm saying?

The majority of people are perfectly okay with living this way and that's great; they have found what they want. But I wasn't happy. I didn't want to wait until I was 65 and retire and have a certain amount of money which would then allow me to do whatever the hell I want. For far too long, I've expected less of myself; I sold myself short. I wasted so many years of my life not even trying to follow my own path, and that, along with other traumas in my life, chipped away at me mentally until I was so far removed from living the life I wanted, that I was lost.

Neil's Notes

Let's have a little fun here.

If I ask you, what is the one thing you would like more than anything else in this life? What would it be? For me, I would love to travel the world promoting my new movie, for which I was nominated for four Academy Awards, best actor, best director, best writer, and best film.

Far-fetched? Possibly. Not achievable? Maybe.

But it's my dream. I can dream whatever I want. Nobody needs to know. I go to sleep with this thought, and as I drift off to sleep, I find myself adding new elements each night, with a huge smile on my face.

What is your dream?

When you're in bed, run it through your mind.

Dream often. Dream big. Dream tonight.

—◆—

Chapter 4
Is there a future?

I could see NO Future.

Is there a future in this life for you? Can you see a future for yourself? Or maybe it's just something you haven't thought about. But what if you did? If you sat down and thought about your future. What would it look like? It's a difficult task at the best of times, one which I feel we often neglect to consider. As I thought 'que sera, sera' to myself, I was sure I had no future, as I knew my 'whatever will be, will be' was death.

For so long, I had no purpose or real direction for my life. It seemed to me that I was going around in circles, day after day, week after week, and year after year, not knowing where I was headed. My depression and anxiety made sure of this uncertainty, while instilling within me a belief that only one thing was certain: That as long as I lived, I would continue to suffer, to remain stuck in this deep dark rut. That is, until I worked up the courage to release myself – forever!

It seemed to me that I did not 'get' life.

I thought I was the only one with this feeling, unsure what it meant to live a life, while everyone else moved forward, without me. Nothing I did helped me to shake this feeling; not the excitement of starting a new job, moving to live in a new location, or even the joy of a holiday. There was always something dragging me down. Nothing

I ever did seemed like progress. Not buying a house, not completing two bloody degrees; nothing. It felt as if everyone was in on some big secret, about how to move on in life, and how to live it well, but that secret was being kept from me.

With me being so lost and uncertain in this life, I have so many 'lost' years. I feel now, even though I'm in my 40's, that I'm still stuck in my late teens to early 20's, too young to settle down and marry, and not ready to have children. I'm still finding my feet and exploring the direction of my life in every aspect. I'm not sure if this makes sense, but because my depression and anxiety had control over me for so long, I never really lived. I didn't live up to whatever potential I possessed, if any. I hadn't done what all others in their 20's had done, maybe travelling the world, experiencing new cultures. I hadn't done what those in their 30's had done, maybe build a career and a home.

I know it doesn't sound very logical but it's a feeling which at times still sits with me and has caused me to believe I'm so far behind the rest of you that I will never catch up, never experience what life truly has to offer; that I will never shake off this feeling of missing out; that I will remain in this limbo forever.

This was blocking my future.

I was stuck because of that continuous masking of my mental health problems. Having those problems blocked my path towards living the life I wanted. I didn't feel ready to step forward in life as many of my friends have, to take on more responsibility. I didn't feel ready to move on with certain elements of my life, and I wondered if I would ever be ready and mature enough to do so?

Like, at the time of writing, I'm not married and have not really been in a serious relationship for twelve or so years. I have no kids, and I'm not sure if I want any. If marriage and children are milestones of adulthood, then will I ever become an adult? Don't get me wrong, it's not that I don't want to grow up, or that I have a fear of growing old, but I feel that if I accept the stage of life I'm at now and follow what society expects of me, then I will miss out even more than I already have. Yes, it's true that we should all embrace each season and stage of our lives, but we should each do it in our own way.

And maybe me believing I had no future stems from not having this 'personalised' purpose. I've tried and tested many avenues: I have studied a sports degree, worked as a youth worker, a sports development officer, worked in community development, set up my own fitness business, studied law, studied for the bar exams and so on. But each time, I never felt satisfied with any of those pursuits. I would find myself going down one avenue and stopping, then trying another and stopping. Always start, stop, start, stop. Never being able to follow through.

Yes, of course, the lack of a sense of purpose in my life played a massive part in this. Why should I commit to anything concrete or explore any avenue, when I knew I wasn't going to be around to follow it through? So, I allowed myself to plod along in the so-called comfort zone, waiting for the inevitable.

Do you have a purpose or some direction in your life?

I felt it was too late for me. My friends were all moving on and doing well – jobs, family, fully informed of their chosen direction – but I was being left behind. During one counselling session we explored my sense of feeling lost in this life, that I did not have a place here, had nothing to look forward to, and could not be excited about anything that might lie ahead.

The counselling sessions over the previous few months really helped me explore and find solutions to many problems, but I still felt this hole, like something was missing. That lost feeling, no excitement about life, and life boring me as I moved aimlessly through each day.

And that was it. I was moving aimlessly through life, staying safe and not pursuing some future for myself. After the eye-opening exploratory discussion with my counsellor, it dawned on me that I needed to have a purpose of my own. That I actually could have a purpose which was mine, meaningful to me. It did not have to follow the rules which I perceived society was setting for us – 9-5 job, marriage, kids. It could be whatever I goddamn well wanted it to be.

So, what does this mean for you? It means you can explore options and find things which are purposeful or meaningful that YOU want for your life. It can be whatever you want it to be! The only criteria being, you need to find a thing that excites you, one that makes you smile, that you want to wake up for each morning. Something you connect to personally but which also allows you to connect with others. This something gives you satisfaction; it makes you feel proud and full. It will be a struggle, but a struggle you chose and something which makes sense in your life right now.

I want to help myself and manage my mental health problems, and in turn I want to help others. One such way I'm doing this is by writing this book. Another way I do this is by setting up a business in mental health and wellbeing. Exploring your purpose can be fun. As they say, the sky's the limit.

Start off by asking yourself some questions about your current situation. Are you working a job you hate? If so, why are you still in it? Is it enough to just do it for the money? Are you doing the college course you want to? Are you just continuing because it's good to have a degree, even though you might have wasted four years you might have put to better use?

Be open to change.

Know that you can change at any stage in your life, no matter your age. Hey, look at me. I changed at 40 years of age. I'm not married, don't have kids, and I don't own a house anymore. I probably don't fit the 'expected' profile of a 40-year-old man, but who gives a fuck. I'm now doing my own thing. Don't let wrong or past decisions in your early life dictate your future. You can always change; it's your life after all.

And don't get misguided by other people's purpose.

My brother Paul has a wife and four kids, a business and a nice house. He is, by any measure, quite a successful man. Should a house, a wife, children and a successful business be my purpose? No! You don't have to emulate others' successes, because their purpose in life is not yours. That is his, not mine. My friends are married with kids and live in nice houses in towns more suited for families. Should that be my purpose as well? No? That's theirs. Coming to the realisation that I could choose my own purpose or meaning in life really liberated me, opening me up to new possibilities and a new way of looking at life.

Should I?

As discussed, having no purpose or direction was a factor in why I felt lost for so many years. Another contributory factor is one I've touched on before; that society makes us believe there is a path we *should* follow, and if we don't, we are different. It dangles the carrot for us to follow in the same footsteps as those who have gone before, and entices us to stay on the same path as those around us today:

Go to school and we will reward you with a college place.

Go to college and we will reward you with a job.

Get married, buy a house, have kids, work for a few decades, then retire and we will offer you some nice rewards along the way.

This might vary, but for most people the path is more or less the same. This suits some people. If that's you, then fine! Follow that path to the best of your ability.

But that's NOT what I wanted.

It wasn't easy to accept the realisation that I wanted something different for my life. Accepting it meant I stood out even further from the crowd. It felt as if I was doing something wrong. It made me constantly question myself as to why I had to be so awkward? Why the hell can't I just be normal like everyone else? They all enjoy life (but do they, really?) and are getting on with it, so what the fuck is wrong with me? I should be just like them, right?

After that explorative counselling session, I felt a little more at ease as I realised that it's okay for me to want different things for my life. I don't have to compare my life, my wants, my desires or my vision for my future to anybody else's. It's my life, and I can walk whichever path I choose. I often hear people say, 'I don't have a choice'. Well, I'm here today to tell you, YES YOU DO! We all have a choice and, in fact, not making a choice IS a choice.

So, I implore you to make the choice today to find YOUR purpose. That means putting yourself and your feelings first for a change. This will benefit you and all those connected to you in the long term.

You don't have to be constrained by the choices you made when you were 18 years old, or by the course you studied in college. (Hey, I studied for two degrees; sports degree and a law degree, totalling nine years of college, and I don't work in either area.) You don't even have to bow to the pressure of being expected to take over the family business. If I had kept on the path which was laid for me by my decisions when I was 18, then I would not be as progressed in my state of good mental health as I'm today. I would, without question, still be clouded by darkness and consumed by anxiety.

If something doesn't feel right to you then question it.

Why does it not feel right for you? What can you do about it? Find out, then do it! Do not be stuck on a path others think you should be travelling. They are not you; they don't have to live in your shoes each and every day.

Neil's Notes

Hey, I have an idea. Put down the book (only for a few mins, mind), and have a think about what your ideal future would look like. Ah, go on, give it a try!

Here are some questions to help you:

1. Where would you live? In a house? Apartment? Do you own it?
2. Do you drive in this ideal future? What kind of car?
3. Are you married? Single? Partner?
4. Do you have a kid? How many? Boys or girls?
5. Where are you working? For a company? For yourself?
6. What hobbies do you have? Writing? Reading? Running?
7. Do you play an instrument?
8. What else do you see in your future?

So have a real think about it, go mad, have fun! Dream and plan big! Guess what? The thing is, this fun activity can become your reality. It has for me.

I do this in the form of a vision board, every year. This is an amazing tool you can use to focus on what you TRULY want out of life. It consists of a collage of magazine cut-outs, pictures, phrases, and words that represent the kind of life you want to live in the future.

This could include your fitness levels, professional success, travel, cars, homes, and any other experiences you would like to integrate into your life. It truly is a powerful tool; one I know will keep me focused on achieving and moving forward. But it also reminds me that I now have a life and a future, just like everyone else. I'm not different, I'm not 'not normal', I just want different things.

If you're lost or feeling left behind then STOP!

Please take action and explore your purpose for this stage of your life. And, YES, YOU HAVE ONE! We all do, because remember what I said, your purpose or your point is whatever YOU want it to be right now! Please believe me. LIVE LIFE, and live YOUR WAY, find how to live purposefully and with meaning.

I would highly recommend you making your own vision board. Be creative and have fun and fill it with pictures which mean something to you and your vision for the future. Hang it up somewhere you'll see it every day. Mine is in my bedroom.

—◆—

Chapter 5
Wait! There's more

Am I liked?

This is a tough one. There are no two ways about it, this is bloody tough. Imagine questioning whether people like you. Each and every time you meet new people, as well as wondering whether those in your life right now genuinely care.

All I ever wanted was to be accepted by others. I felt like an outsider so many times in my life. Even now in my forties I can still feel this way. I get the sense that people just don't like me, that I'm not their 'cup of tea', as we say. I've always felt like the outsider to the 'in-gang'.

The majority of the time, I'm sure this notion of not being liked is just a result of my overthinking, a concept I have conjured up for some reason or another. The problem is, it has been ingrained over many years. Which makes change difficult. Whether it's true or not, believing it has caused me to detach myself from others, even those I know. This is the self-doubt, lack of confidence and self-hate that depression and anxiety bring with it. If you don't like anything about yourself, why the hell would anybody else?

Looking back on years gone by, I know I've tried too hard to be accepted and that was mainly down to the fact that I was masking my mental health problems. I felt that I had to distract people's attention away from what was really going on inside my head. Very often my go-to deflection method, if in a group setting, would be to make myself the centre of attention; become the joker, the class-messer, try to make others laugh, thereby dismissing any suspicions they might be harbouring.

I became that student; the clown in school who'd get into trouble for disrupting the smooth running of the class. If I could make my classmates laugh, then I hoped they would think I was okay, someone they would like to hang out with. The whole time I was clowning, I still never really believed people liked me all that much. The paradox of being the clown was that I felt people never considered me friend-material and so would not invite me to hang out.

As a kid all you want is to be included. Kids often count the number of friends they have. As adults we know the number is of no importance, and declines as we advance in age, and change location and interests. Those who usually remain friends in adulthood are true friends, relationships which would be hard to replace. If only I had known, while growing up, that numbers mean nothing.

This feeling of not being wanted is something I've tried to suppress and forget about. It's also something I desperately didn't want others to know about as I felt it would have a knock-on effect, deterring others from befriending me. Who wants people to know they are not liked?

Time and again I would question, to myself, why people didn't like me. Maybe it was because I tried too hard, maybe it was because I was just a dick, or maybe I wasn't interesting, or maybe it was my name (Kelders not being an Irish name). What the hell was it?

For all the cheeky trouble I got into, I don't think there was any badness in me. I do believe I'm a good person. I listen intently to people when they speak. I take people's problems on board and help them as much as possible, sometimes even neglecting my own wants and needs. All the traits of being a good friend, or so I thought.

I wanted to fit in and be included, just like everyone else, but looking back, there were many times I was left out of activities or events by so-called friends. I suppose you could say that they were friends when it suited them. As a kid that hurts. Hell, as an adult it doesn't get much easier, especially if you're so unsure of yourself and in constant confusion as to why you bloody exist. Then, to me, this exclusion felt like yet another rejection.

The good news is, although I can't change being accepted or befriended, I can change my reaction to the situation. First of all, I learned how to be comfortable with myself, in my own space. Then I learned to be okay with boredom, and learned how to find ways to amuse myself. If we can become comfortable on our own and in our own space, if we strive to become the type of person who has the motivation to keep active, regardless of company, we become less reliant on others and spend less time seeking acceptance.

I've also learned to accept that not everyone in this life will like me, and I don't need everyone to like me. Not everyone will be looking to make friends, and that's okay. It's not a reflection on me; there might be other reasons for this, to which I'm not privy.

I'm more secure in my own skin and now don't need to seek out other people's approval. Yes, of course it's nice and feels good when we meet new people and forge new friendships and gain that sense of acceptance but as they say: I am my own man.

Over the last six or seven years I've really worked on myself and my personal development. Now, I can say that I kinda like myself, and know I deserve better than to be badly treated by anyone. I'm positive that there are people out there who will like me for who I am, and for what I can bring to the table. Those are words I never thought I would hear coming out of my mouth. But that's the power of believing in yourself, and working hard to find a way out of the mist.

It has progressed a step further and I'm at the stage where I'm now confident enough to choose who I want as part of my life. I'm more aware of how people make me feel when around them. I also became aware that when in certain people's company, I had to act differently, to not be myself, which, in turn, does not make me feel good about myself. Those people I have removed, and am the better for it.

Trying to fit in with this or that group has always been part of my life. Changing from my true self to fit in, to and please others, or put my own feelings aside to avoid troubling others.

When in a group where alcohol was in full flow, I would often take on the role of the joker, the messer, trying to make everyone laugh. When full of alcohol this role was easy, natural and enjoyable.

Many years later, when trying to find out who I was and who I wanted to be, I realised I actually hated this part of me, and decided to actively change it. I'm happy to tell you I've done so but... yeah, there's a but... While in Cyprus, and during the initial stages of meeting new people, I found myself consuming alcohol, and once again becoming the joker of the pack. It wasn't necessarily a bad thing. The guys were good fun and, if I'm honest, it did gain me acceptance to the group. I do have good friends here, but this reflex action, which I seem compelled to resort to, just reminded me of times, when I previously felt I had let myself down.

I had worked so hard to change this. But still I felt the need to resort to a mask of sorts to be accepted. I wasn't as confident as I had led myself to believe. I reverted back to joker Neil, afraid to reveal the real me and be okay with it. I would truly prefer people to take me as I am or don't take me at all, rather than be the dancing monkey. So, I still have work to do. I know I always will if I want to stay true to myself.

It is possible to find positives in every situation. On the upside I was very aware of how I acted, and the feeling behind it, so I set about, once again, working at changing. I took a break from the Friday, after-work drinking culture. When ready, I gradually reintroduced myself to the setting, but on more stable terms.

I have a few beers, have a laugh and enjoy the banter. I'm not the last to leave the party, but call it a day after three beers or before midnight. This is more within my control and I still get to experience the buzz of the night and connect with new friends.

Now I find myself meeting up with the group at the beach or for a house party or a night out. It doesn't seem to have affected their view of me one bit. Wow, wow, wow! If I had bloody known this over twenty years ago! But hey, we live and learn; or at least, we should live and learn. As they say: Better late than never.

Today I find myself able to walk away from situations which don't feel right. I don't give it a second thought and I feel empowered by doing so. I no longer fall over myself trying to change other people's view of me. I just move on. Being comfortable with yourself (which we touch on, later), and being able to walk away from these situations, is so liberating. It has led to me being able to walk away, not just in many social situations, but also work situations and jobs when I felt there was no other recourse because my health was suffering.

Left outside

I've had countless occasions when things were just plain shit. I've had those 'friends' who, for some reason or other, would not include me in certain fun activities, but then seemed to be all about me when it suited them. Over the years this has caused me pain, distress, questioning and plain old sadness. Is this something you can relate to? Being left out and feeling not wanted?

When in secondary school, Friday nights were a big social occasion. Friends would plan to meet in town that night and just hang out. I wouldn't be invited, and I would never be the type to just invite myself. They would chat and plan it in front of me and not one of them would think to ask me if I was going; that hurt. How could these guys who I hung out with and share a laugh with, be so cruel? I would find myself sitting at home, alone, on Friday evening, in front of the TV, trying not to think about what was happening outside of the walls of my house. Trying not to think about the fun my 'friends' were having. Trying not to think that they were not giving me a second thought. All the time aware that I would hear it being discussed over the coming days. As I sat there in the darkness of our 'good' sitting room, I could feel myself being pounded by thoughts encouraging me to slide into a never-ending well of darkness which would become all too familiar as the years passed by.

There were many times when a close friend would arrange a night of cards with our group and, again, I would never be invited. We would be hanging out days later and they would be recounting stories of incidents that happened on that 'great' night. Again, in bloody front of me. I often wonder what was going through their minds. Did they just not give a fuck? Why did they pick and choose when to hang out with me? If they hated me so much then why not just tell me to get lost, right?

It hurt so badly not to be included. This, too, fed into my mental health problems. It was hard. It made me question yet again as to why

I was so different? What was wrong with me? Was I that hard to like?

To this day I hate to hear of kids, or adults for that matter, being bullied or feeling alone. I know what it's like. Hand on heart, it's one of the worst feelings in the world, to be on the outside. To feel nobody gives a shit about you, to not be liked, to believe you would not be missed. As I write this, I can feel the emotion building and more memories of being excluded are beating like a drum against my head.

Such experiences have an effect on you. I became very insecure, it dented my confidence, drove me further into my darkness, distanced me from people, made me awkward in new situations, and created a block to connecting or opening myself up to people. It was another area added to the growing list for me to work on.

I think I can safely say that we all just want to be included, to be liked, to feel part of something. I'm of the belief that life is made a whole lot better when we connect with people. Events, activities and experiences are all the better for it.

So, if you can do one thing when you finish reading this book, then let it be this: Invite someone to something. Chat to someone. Check in on someone and include someone. For you it might be a small gesture, to them it will mean the world. I know it would have meant the world to me!

Neil's Notes

Of course, putting yourself out there to connect with others can be very daunting. It often heightened my anxiety. As already mentioned, I do believe there were times when it was all in my head, this not being liked by people.

If I did not receive a call or text from someone, then I knew it was because they must not care. When in a stronger frame of mind, I questioned this and found out something interesting: I did not text or call them either. Was I too precious to send them a message or ask them to hang out? Why should they have to be the ones to make the first move?

I would convince myself that there was no point in making contact as this friend or that would not reply. They will reject any ideas I put forward. I would get so worked up that any action I wanted to take would be shot down

Do you find that you never initiate a message? Or organise a group of friends to meet? Do you think your friend(s) are not messaging because they don't want to hang out? You're only guessing right? You can't say for sure. The only way you'll truly find an answer is by biting the bullet and putting yourself out there.

Give it a try. Message a friend.

Before you send it, you need to accept a few things. For one, they might not message back straight away, so don't sit with phone in hand checking it every five minutes. They might decline your offer, and give an excuse as to why. That excuse is valid as far as you're concerned, okay? So don't speculate otherwise. You can do this!

—◆—

Chapter 6
The gift that keeps on giving

I just want to sleep! Depression and anxiety disrupted all aspects of my life and sleep, or should I say the lack of it, was no different. I craved a night where I could just slide into bed, close my eyes and be woken by the sunlight filtering into my room. We can all dream, I suppose. My sleep reality was a very different story; instead of feeling refreshed from a night of sleep, I was left drained by the lack of. Most nights I was hitting a whopping forty-five minutes sleep per night. This is no fun, believe me. I would be exhausted, but once I hit the sack, my mind would go into overdrive with thoughts swirling through my head, my eyes wide open. I just lay tossing and turning, frustrated to the point of tears, craving the shut-eye needed to be able to function at some level the next day.

No such luck. The day would begin with a struggle. Exhausted, I would have to rip myself from my bed and get on. Then I would doze off at intervals during the day. A good – or bad – example that springs to mind, depending on which way you look at it, is the night before my first day at the co-working space in Cyprus. Concerns over how the day would pan out consumed me, creating the usual sensations of overwhelm. I envisaged each step I would take the next day: Walking up to the building, walking in through the doors and on entering the building, every person silently working at their desk would automatically lift their heads and focus in on me, the stranger.

I liken this to a scene in a movie where we see the new prisoner walking with the prison guards to his cell and other inmates hissing and jeering him. A total over-exaggeration, I know, but in my overactive mind it's not. As I stand in the office space, sweat drips down my bald head and soaks my grey tee-shirt as their laser eyes follow me to a seat at one of the hot desks. As I sit quietly at my desk, afraid to turn my head left or right, I hear chatter and laughter behind me. All the other co-workers enjoy a coffee and some banter. While, once again, I am the outsider sitting alone. Probably being the butt of their jokes…

This scenario I told myself created a fear and apprehension that caused me to lie exhausted in bed, staring into nothingness, on the verge of convincing myself to not go into the co-working space the next day. That is incredible if you think about it. Something that has not happened. Something which more than likely will not happen has this control over me. I was trying to convince myself to avoid this 'inevitable' suffering by not going into the co-working space at all. Which, may I add, was one of the main reasons for my brave decision to move to Cyprus in the first place. Crazy, right! Talk about self-sabotage. Because I know that if I don't meet people and get out of my house, I will struggle greatly with my mental health. The thing is, you and I do this, time and again, creating these fictional scenarios which block us from taking back control of our lives. We become a prisoner of our own thoughts.

Imagine the effect this lack of sleep has on one's body. This was my life for years on end, never getting unbroken sleep. I just couldn't function properly. It would feed my mood for the day and create a body in a constant state of fatigue. It got to the stage, which scared me a little, when one morning I 'awoke', having got shut-eye for forty-five minutes, which of course usually happened close to the time my alarm would sound off. I opened my eyes to my body shaking uncontrollably as I attempted to get out of bed. I was totally exhausted, as anxiety wasn't just plaguing my mind, but my body, too, crushing me down to a severe low.

This became my new norm. I called it the 'Iceland effect', likening it to a constant state of near twenty-four hours daylight. At all times being wide awake. But time does not stop and morning moves into afternoon and onto evening time and me in my exhausted state needs to keep plodding away; regardless of the battle which brews inside; anxious, low, stressed and worried.

I had to do something. This had to be addressed. I could not go on like this for much longer. I craved, like Hamlet, to sleep, a chance for some peace. It was impacting my life as a whole. When morning came around, I often found myself texting clients to cancel sessions (I had a fitness business) as I lay deflated with an incoming low in bed, which after some time would change to me being more anxious and overwhelmed because I had let my clients down, I failed them. The message or, should I say, the lie I sent to clients would be at an hour of the night when I knew it would not be seen until morning. The lie was one about my condition, usually texting I had been sick during the night, never revealing the true reason. What could I do to turn this continuous cycle around? Was there anything that could be done?

I took a look at my sleeping patterns and analysed my morning routine. Ever since I was a child I would wake early. I loved to have the mornings to myself. When I was a kid, I would wake early and watch some old black and white movies such as Tarzan or Zulu (I loved them). I still wake early; this has never changed. I don't think it ever will and to be honest I do enjoy being up early. It gives me a comfort as I feel I have the world to myself.

I then took a look at my evening routine. More often than not I would fall asleep on the couch with the TV on, but be wide awake at bedtime. I needed a better routine to wind down my day, and a big part of this was to turn off my electronics. I know. Obvious, right? But true.

I set about exploring better sleep and what worked and didn't work for me. I now have a routine which suits me but, of course, is open to being adapted when needed. The first thing I do is wind down my evening. I drink some chamomile tea and spray some lavender oil onto my pillow. I'm in bed with a book by 10pm, with the alarm set to prompt me to turn out the light, by 10.30pm.

These few natural additions to my sleep routine have helped, but, of course, at times I neglect this new routine, when I feel really good and on top of things, and everything is going well for me. This maintenance stage is very important, and one I need to keep on top of. If not, then I fall back into my old patterns, lacking sleep, lacking energy, and lacking the want to live. Drastic, I know, but true. There is always a solution and the best place to start is with yourself.

How long more?

Have you any idea how hard it is to live with depression? Those lows, that total lack of energy and that darkness which just engulfs you? It's absolutely soul-destroying because you know the beginning, middle and end. With each episode, you know the impending doom that lies ahead. You know you'll be thrown into a turbulent darkness, naked as the day you were born. If and when you come through that, there's little reprieve, as your mind is already focused in anticipation on the next bout, which you know is incoming, though you're uncertain as to when, where or how it will hit.

Oh, silly me, I almost forgot! Just to make sure you don't get a handle on things, some of us experience a bout of anxiety before or after the depressive episode. And let me tell you this is no picnic. To lose control of body and mind, while failing to see a way of gaining back some of this control, is frightening. Anxiety is sneaky. One minute all is okay, the next bang – overwhelmed, fearful, worried, and sweating buckets. Like its cousin, depression, it consumes both body and mind, not letting you rest for a second. Everything seems to be a trigger, with no perceivable way out and, like a depressive episode, you just have to wait until it's ready to release you.

I recall one Thursday morning, 10th September, 2015 (I know because I've written many of my experiences down). It was 7.30 am, and I found myself sitting in the kitchen in darkness. My head was spinning. I just couldn't relax. The walls were caving in on me. My negative thoughts were on rapid fire. I sat there, defeated, thinking, *It Gets Harder Every Fucking Day and I Don't Know How Long More I Can Handle!*

But what I did know was that I needed to act right away. I knew all too well what this overwhelming mess of confusion and self-doubt could do to me if I just sat there and let it work its potential. Everything gets on top of me. I mean EVERYTHING. My beard frustrates me, and my hair. I haven't shaved my head in three days, and the little bit that does grow makes me feel and look like a sixty-year-old man. Work, even though it's the weekend, consumes my thoughts. The fact that I'm behind, the upcoming meetings I've scheduled for next week. So many thoughts just going on and on and on....

Okay! Action needed NOW! I initiate a little self-talk – 'Time to get out. Get up and out of the house. Change the setting. Go NOW into the bathroom.'

I shaved my head and beard. I'm in my mother's house in Kerry. I inform her what's going on, and that I need some time to myself to sort it. I reassure her, so as not to worry her. I'm very anxious now. As I eye my weak self in the mirror, I'm disgusted at what stares back at me. Okay, enough, 'I'm outta here'. I pack my gym bag, and collect my laptop so as to have options available. I can either go to the gym (but today is my rest day) and/or I can write some words. I know writing helps, and if I write about this event, what is happening to me now, this morning's anxiety, it will initiate my calming process and hopefully I can claw back the day. Usually, this level of anxiety would sink me and my day would be a total wipe-out.

I head for a local café to get a table in a quiet corner, hoping nobody will stop to chat, and write. I am able to get my thoughts on paper quickly. I'm sitting in the café breathing and focusing. Okay, I'm more relaxed and starting to calm. My thoughts are clearer, calmer and, more importantly, logical. NO! IT DOES NOT GET HARDER EVERY FUCKING DAY and YES, I KNOW I CAN HANDLE IT.

This episode was the first time I really got a handle on my anxiety. Usually, it would consume me and I would just try to ride it out, not knowing how long it would last. A day, two or maybe three? This time, I stopped sitting in it. I took action, made choices, and kept moving forward all day. When I was going through the anxiety, there was no time to analyse it. I just needed to address it as best I could in order to give myself some relief. I'm proud of the action I had undertaken, even though it took until later that evening to ground myself fully. But it was a win for me for sure, as this could have gone on much longer.

Another positive from that day was that I was also able to open up to my mother and calmly explain how I was feeling. Informing her of the steps I needed to take, and that I was okay to do this alone. This opening up to her would mean less worry for the both of us. The combination of each of those small steps allowed me to win back my day.

When I go through a bout of depression or anxiety, I try to reflect on the event. To explore some potential triggers and also pinpoint the steps I took which helped alleviate this anxiety. I also looked at those which did not work so well. On this occasion, I realise I'd had a very poor night's sleep. A trigger for sure. I'm worried when visiting my mother, in case she might notice the turmoil rumbling on inside my human frame. I try to ensure that my mood doesn't dip, or I become overwhelmed. This pressure, which I put on myself, is a contributing factor. The triggers build up until I can hide it no more. I'm gone! You can see how it's like a domino effect. Each thought triggers another, and then another, and so on, until both my body and mind seem to be out of control.

This Thursday, 10th September, the little steps I integrated into my morning helped me claw back the day, because four hours later I have restored some calmness. In previous months I would become so worked-up and so far gone, that my day would be lost. I'd probably be stuck to the bed not sleeping, not resting, but recycling thought after thought, sapping every last ounce of energy, hoping it would not feed into tomorrow.

Nowadays, I'm more in tune with myself and what I need to do when certain experiences occur. This is something I've learned through trial and error. Having gone through experiences like this many times I now know the steps I need to take to bring me back. Steps to win back my day. I'm also aware that I will have to adapt or progress these steps as time goes by, and not rest on my laurels.

Neil's Notes

Does anxiety arrive at your door? What, if anything, have you learned that helps you to manage it?

Don't become complacent, and make sure you keep searching and finding new ways that will help you. To help you achieve this, I want to share some of the steps I took that day in 2015.

1. I changed my location by getting out of the house.
2. I walked to the cafe, rather than drive, which had me out in the fresh air and was a distracting activity.
3. I carved out time alone for the process (you might want to talk to someone).
4. I treated myself to a cappuccino and a scone.
5. I listened to music that recalled some happy memories.
6. Once I was ready, I wrote about the day's experience. Getting on paper helps to address the situation. I find that writing relieves the intense pressure I feel in my head.
7. I thought about why I might have become anxious and what I could do the next time it happens.
8. Keep physically active – even though it was my rest day from training, I did some light exercise. Exercise allows me to be present and focus.

Depression and anxiety can overpower us without warning. I'm thankfully aware of this danger now and able to actively do something about it (as above). D & A don't have to set the tone for my day or week. I can gradually ground myself.

The beauty about this is, that if I can, well so can you.

You've got this!

—◆—

Depression and anxiety also physically consumed me!

There is no getting away from either depression or anxiety. When they hit, they hit hard, no holds barred. They're like that terrible house-mate who invades your physical space, while also getting into your head. There's no let-up whatsoever and they consume you to the point of exhaustion.

Fatigue, frustration, and anger would penetrate my whole body, stop me in my tracks, as I didn't know why it was triggered or how to deal with it. There was this one time I was trying to get back to running in order to help myself with a very low mood. I set off on my run and as I was moving along the road, I felt my head being infiltrated by this heavy feeling, inside and out. Best described as this dark fog closing in to smother my skull and brain.

A few years ago, there was an ad on Irish TV for a charity called Concern. It described how people in Kenya were having issues with blindness. To illustrate this point of blindness we see the screen gradually goes black. This ad, for me, demonstrated how my smothered brain feels. It's as if my brain sets out all bright and light but gradually would begin to narrow, causing an increased dark heaviness.

You might not experience depression like a darkness smothering your brain, but this is just one of many ways I feel it physically.

Another bizarre way that I've used to describe my depression is reference to The Simpsons. If you've ever watched The Simpsons, you'll be aware of the cartoon Bart and Lisa loved to watch called The Itchy and Scratchy Show. A cartoon featuring a cat (Scratchy) and his enemy a blue mouse (Itchy), an obvious parody of Tom & Jerry.

In almost every episode, Scratchy is killed, or at least brutally injured, by Itchy. In one episode I recall the blue mouse brutally killed the cat by drilling him with lead, you know, shooting him with a tommy gun (it was 1920's mobster style killing). What happened when Scratchy was shot is that we saw the blood drained from his body through the bullet holes in his toes. THAT is how my depression would feel sometimes.

As if my body was draining of blood and life through holes in my toes. I could feel it physically, totally drained of all feelings.

These are some of the descriptive ways a depressive episode would feel when shutting me down and cutting me off from life and all feeling. It's all consuming, all powerful and with a feeling of no escape. Ever!

I had to find ways to overcome this darkness. There are many things I've tried and tested, to help shine some light when my depression hit. Mostly I would try to distract my mind and become more present in what I was doing at any given moment.

Neil's Notes

What I will now share with you can be done anywhere, by anyone. Take driving as an example. If I'm driving and I feel that low period setting in, I try to focus on things within my immediate environment. I see something, I name it by speaking out in a strong, loud voice. 'Oh, there is a red light, a black sign, a brown jacket.' I do this for a minute, or two or three, and then I advance it (you will find your mind wandering, so when that happens just refocus on the world around you).

Then I do the same again but this time I call something by a different name. For example, I start off by seeing a red sign, I don't say it out loud yet, but keep searching for something else to see. I see a green bike, so this time instead of calling it a green bike I call it a red sign (which I had seen just before the bike). Then the next thing I see, for example a yellow car, I call this yellow car, green bike. The goal here is to have my brain working hard and distracting my mind even further.

Give it a try now. As I said it can be done anywhere at any time, so if you're in your sitting room, then look around you and start naming things. Better again, get off your seat and walk around while doing it. Follow my advice in the above paragraphs.

Distract that mind today!

—◆—

Chapter 7
Am I the only one?

It felt as if I was the only one going through this pain, this struggle, this uncertainty. The constant lows and highs, the nagging want for it to end by any means possible. As I looked around me, everyone was coasting through life, not a care in the world. I was the only one in my family, my circle of friends, my town, my country, heck probably the world dealing with this pain. As I was the only person alive suffering like this, it meant I would have to deal with it alone. I mean who could I ask for help and support? Nobody would understand what I'm going through. If I did let them see inside this head of mine, I would come across as odd, different, be shunned and very much an outsider. I needed to face my reality. I'm a lone sufferer. I alone have to deal with it. This interpretation of my situation isolated me from all of you and created a deep loneliness inside. A deep, dark, empty loneliness. I just got a shiver as I wrote this. It's a feeling or situation I never want to experience again. It's feels as if there is absolutely no way out of it. Rock bottom!

Of course, I now know that I wasn't the only one going through these struggles. I, also now know that opening up to others exposes a more real, better-informed version of myself, allowing me to under- stand there are many more people out there, struggling with their own pain, also, feeling alone, isolated and removed.

Maybe someone next to you right now. I can almost guarantee that someone you know very well is struggling in some way right at this moment, as you read these words. Think about that!

Can you think of someone else who has a mental health condition? Are you finding it difficult to identify someone? Have you thought about all the areas of mental health including; depression, anxiety, stress, addiction, ADHD, some forms of autism. Yes? No? Did you know they are all classified as mental health conditions, according to the World Health Organisation?

Did you know that twenty percent of the world population at any given time will experience mental health problems? That's 1 in 5 people and if we work the maths, it means we all should know someone in our lifetime, or we already have known someone who has gone through one of those problems or conditions. So, let me tell you right now, there is no way you're alone in this suffering or unique in your suffering. There are more of us out there just like you. I'm like you and you're like me!

Then, if you're not unique in this suffering, you're not alone in all the experiences and emotions this suffering generates. This, in turn, means there are others out there who will understand exactly what you go through. If you allow yourself the chance to talk to someone and open up, you'll find that you're not the lone sufferer in this world. You'll find people wanting to help you. So, listen to me: You don't have to fight this battle alone. Once you open up, disclose your inner battles to someone, and seek help, this feeling of loneliness, sadness, of not being connected, will begin to dissipate.

Even though being physically alone and the emotion of being lonely are very different, I believe they feed off each other, and gain momentum, like a hamster wheel, until you feel there is no way to get off, and you're spiralling further and further into your darkness. The simple step of opening up about what is going on inside that head of yours will also have a knock-on effect, spiralling you towards brighter times; moving you away from this darkness, counteracting the loneliness, and allowing for the human need of connecting.

The mask is not your friend

As my struggles continued, I felt myself drifting further away from people, interacting less. When I did interact, I had created a barrier so not to have my struggles exposed. As I have mentioned, this created a deep loneliness within, which is not only present when I'm alone with my thoughts, but also when out with other human beings.

I have felt very lonely during times which should have been pure celebration. At Christmas time, being surrounded by up to sixteen family members. When with a partner, or when out with friends. Not that you would ever have guessed, as I hid this darkness by being the life and soul of the party. Loneliness for me comes down to not being connected to others which triggers such a feeling of a deep sadness and emptiness, I feel removed from others both physically and mentally.

I know this feeling all too well and is one I don't want others to feel. It does not have to be this way for you. You can change this too; you can remove yourself from loneliness. But this has to involve you taking some action. It's possible for each of us to help others move away from their loneliness by simply giving them our time. This might be as simple as checking in with them in person or by call.

As I look back on those lonely times, it dawns on me that maybe it was often created by my own doing. I was the mastermind of my own loneliness. I would decline invitations from friends and family to meet up and go to events, such as weddings and other occasions. I would even decline invitations to meet friends for pints. There are only so many times people will continue to invite you. I mean, how many times does someone like to be rejected? The invites then became few and far between and my sadness and loneliness grew deeper and deeper. It got to the point where I believed nobody gave a fuck about me. At this point I had not yet realised that my constant rejection of their kind offers had led in part to this.

I have been single for many years, since splitting with my long-term girlfriend. Being single made me even more lonely. I wanted to find that special someone, but over the years things never went as I would have hoped, and I've been physically alone. Even though I have a great family, with whom I talk frequently, and friends with whom I meet for the chat, I'm often alone.

In public settings I was masking my problems which was really draining. It was easier to isolate myself at home, deliberately cutting myself off from the outside world; a world I perceived was not for me! Not such a good decision. Putting on this mask seemed to benefit me. It certainly did not allow anyone notice the true me. It had short term 'benefits'. It kept me safe and protected, or so I thought. In reality it was slowly killing me. It was contributing to my mental health problems, not allowing me to face my reality. It only ever covered up the cracks for the very short term. Those cracks were widening beneath this mask on a daily basis. My advice to you is to ditch the mask, face your reality and step forward with the support of others.

As the weeks, months and years passed, I would find myself on my own more and more. Especially as friends moved on with their lives; getting married and having kids. I felt myself becoming more isolated and alone, having that constant feeling of being left behind.

You might ask why I didn't get out and meet people, check out the dating scene? It's not all doom and gloom, don't get me wrong. I did meet people, but I would find it hard to keep up platonic as well as more intimate relationships. I did briefly date some nice women over the years and some others who I should never have gone past the first date with.

It was hard to get out there and join groups and go on dates, though, because I knew I had a lot of problems to deal with, behind the mask. I had convinced myself that I needed to sort myself out before I could take that step. (But sure, I wasn't doing anything to help myself really was I?) I clung to other excuses which prevented me from meeting people; I knew I would not be around this life much longer, so what was the point and why would I create heartache for someone else?

I stayed alone. I stayed within my shell, until I was ready to let people in. You know, after I sorted myself out of course, which again I must reiterate I was DOING NOTHING ABOUT at this point, though I had myself believing that I was doing many things to try to help myself, but that nothing was working. I was beginning to create a distance between myself and friends, not contacting anyone, beginning to spend more time alone. Then my thoughts diverted to thinking that nobody gave a fuck about me. Nobody gives a shit! Which eventually led me to believe, as we have already discussed, that nobody liked me. ASSHOLES!

Now, today, as my understanding of myself and my problems is clearer and my narrative has changed, I realise that I didn't invest time in other people. Back then, I wanted to be alone, in a sense. I wanted for nobody to notice me. Yet deep down, I yearned for connections. I hated that loneliness, I wanted someone in my life, I wanted friends to hang out with. It was fucking hard being alone with those thoughts which were the creators of my loneliness.

Seeking that special someone

Sometimes I tried to connect and come out of my shell, to venture on a date, to find that special someone. Looking back, many of the short-term relationships I did enter into were for all the wrong reasons and many were wrong choices. I entered into relationships I knew deep down would not last. I found myself gravitating towards women and relationships I knew would be difficult to develop; some living in a different part of Ireland, maybe three or so hours away; others living in another country. Some had kids, which would mean a restriction on how often we could meet. There is nothing wrong with any of these life situations, but I think, deep down, I knew when going into the relationship that I didn't want the connection to be anything serious, or last too long.

What I really wanted from them was, I suppose selfishly, to have that feeling of connection, to whatever extent I allowed myself. I wanted to have someone to do things with. I wanted to be able to get in the car or on a plane and go visit them and leave my isolation behind for a few days. I wasn't really aware I was doing this at the time until one day I was having coffee with my good friend, Gráinne. As I chatted about yet another brief relationship and the state of confusion I was in as to why it ended, Gráinne pointed out that it seemed I didn't really want to find a true relationship. I seemed to be allowing myself meet people who, if I really faced up to it, were not for me, that we were at different stages of our life journey.

She was right, so right. I had been doing exactly that. I met people whom I knew I could never have anything long term with and I just plodded along until it ended, not investing anything, being content with the bit of a reprieve it afforded me. When my plodding along became too much for them, they ended it. And get this, even though I knew the relationship was a non-runner from the get-go, when we broke up, I often felt rejected. Yet again nobody wanted me, and I wasn't meant to be with someone. I was destined to be alone. These feelings inevitably led to a low episode.

Obviously, this toying with my own emotions wasn't good for me or my health. But wasn't I, in a way, the instigator of this turbulence? I could not continue like this. It would send me over the edge. I needed to get myself sorted and change my narrative on relationships. I needed to want to meet someone. I needed to be open to more long-term relationships and I also needed to be strong enough to let someone go. If I sense that a relationship isn't good for me, then I need to be able to be open and say so. It wasn't fair on the other people, and it wasn't fair on me to keep the charade going. So, if you think about it, I was partly the source of my own loneliness.

Keeping a relationship going just for the sake of it is not a reason to stay in it. I bet you know someone unhappy in theirs? Or maybe you are, in yours? Neither party ends it because they are afraid of change. Not wanting to hurt someone else, but yet it seems okay for them to be the one who is hurting. Afraid of what people will say. Afraid of being on their own. It's not an easy thing to do, bring a relationship to an end, but sometimes it's the right thing to do. You can come up with a million reasons to stay in it, but I will call bullshit on each one. I myself bought into them all. Looking back, I was a wreck, doing something I didn't want to do. I wasn't living my life. I have the utmost respect for those people who have called off a wedding or have brought a relationship to an end if they truly believe it's not what they want. For me these people are strong, brave and know what they do and, more importantly, do not want. They will end it even though they are fully aware that they will cause great hurt. But I say to you, won't they save everyone from a lot more pain in the future?

Through the years I've had friends come to me for advice. (Oh yeah, true story. I was the guy people would come to for advice; ironic, right?) I could see they were not happy. I would never provide a definitive answer, it's not my place. But I offered my experience and I listened. I waited for the penny to drop as then they were more open to seeing that they had a choice and then realised that they had a decision to make. The ending of a relationship is not a failure, but a realisation that you've both changed and want different things; there is nothing wrong with that.

ALWAYS BE TRUE TO YOURSELF!

If you're wondering: Yes, at the moment I'm still alone. The difference is that now I'm very comfortable with it. As I've stated previously, I've worked on myself and being alone was one of the things I really needed to focus on. That does not mean I'm not open to meeting someone. I would very much like to and I know I will, but I won't force it just to have someone in my life, and I won't settle just for the sake of it. I deserve the best. You do too!

That thing I never talk about

It is true that I'm comfortable on my own. But I haven't been 100% honest with you or, sorry, I mean I haven't opened up to you, fully. I'm presently sitting here in front of my laptop, frozen in fear. I revealed my mental struggles with much openness and honesty, but as I wrote about my turmoil with relationships, I found myself interrupted by thoughts of something else I was hiding behind my mask. Something I thought nobody ever had to know, something I could keep to myself, forever.

But I know now that I should, no, I need to mention this secret problem. I need to address it and talk about it; for my own health. I know, however difficult it is, it will help me. If I don't speak about it, it will eventually give my depression and anxiety some leverage in their mission to knock me down.

This is the first time I will have ever revealed this. You are the first person who will hear this,and know this about me: I am scared. Yeah, I am scared. I'm afraid of what you might think, of what your reaction might be. I'm afraid, because I know my family will read this, and I worry about what they will think. Will they be ashamed of me? Will they be embarrassed that I revealed so much? What will my friends think? What will people I work with think? Will it affect my earning ability? What will women think? Will it be the final nail in my coffin? Neil, single forever. Because let's be honest who wants someone who has mental health issues, and if that were not bad enough, they would have to cope with this further issue, too.

The truth is, I really struggle with sexual intimacy. I am about to experience something which should be exciting, loving; a memorable occasion, but my legs shake uncontrollably, I get a lump in my throat. I try to stop myself from crying.

I feel very alone in this. Am I?

Maybe you have experienced something similar. You may be single and steer clear of intimate encounters, knowing they would be futile to pursue. You long to be intimate, but you know there's no point. Why frustrate yourself, embarrass yourself and make your partner feel undesirable? At least when single we have some control over these intimate needs, but when in a relationship it is not so straight-forward. There are only so many times you can put off the advances of your partner, right?

I wanted to get close to someone and be intimate; this is something all humans want and need. But from the moment I met someone, right up to the time we were to be intimate, I could not get out of my own head. Sometimes I would make it to the bedroom. Things were going fine, I would think to myself, everything was in working order. I would be assessing and thinking this was going to happen; and there in itself lies the problem. The constant thinking, thinking, thinking. Every bloody step of the way. Not being able to enjoy the experience and the moment. In my head all the time. Let's just say, all the blood was rushing from my body to my head. Not good!

I would then become frustrated, annoyed, and stop. "It's okay Neil," she would say. "It's fine, it happens." In my head I'm screaming, shout-ing, calling myself a useless piece of shit. I can't even do this, one of the most natural and beautiful experiences for us humans! "Let's just cuddle," she would add. I don't want to just cuddle, I want to be with you, goddammit! I shouted inside my head. I can't do this anymore. I can't. It kills me. Why is this happening to me? Have I not enough to deal with? I just can't be fully with this beautiful woman, with whom I am very comfortable. I feel terrible for my partner. I have let her down. They say it's okay, but I have just basically rejected her in the worst possible way. This rejection means I don't find her desirable, that she doesn't turn me on. It must feel, to her, as if I am putting her in the dreaded friends' zone. Let me tell you, nothing could be further from the truth. I want this so much. I want to be with her so much.

I tell myself, "No, Neil, this is not okay, she is not okay with this rejection." And I distance myself from intimacy, from relationships, altogether. I shut down. I don't want to make anyone else feel like this, I don't want to let anyone down again. I don't want to hurt someone else, so, instead, choose to hurt myself. I withdraw, and shy away from any form of connection and intimacy, any hope of a loving relationship.

Has this happened to you? Have you put yourself under pressure to perform, wanting so badly to be there with your partner, but no matter what you do, you can't get out of your head and enjoy the moment? You lose the connection, the motion, and just want to curl up and die?

I feared sex. You wonder to yourself how this could ever happen. I mean, it is sex, right? Who doesn't want that? We all do at some stage in our life, am I right? I tried to figure out what was wrong. I did eventually go to my doctor, and stumbled through an explanation of my issue. I said I must be stressed, not mentioning the darkness I was living under. He was very understanding, and suggested that it was a psychological problem or block. We decided I would take Cialis. It worked. Once I got over my fear of meeting someone and being intimate with them, I seemed to have a new lease of life. It worked until... Well, until it didn't. My overthinking made an unwelcome return, the pressure mounted, and once again I was unable to perform. The doctor upped my dosage. Yes, things are happening again, until... You get the picture.

So, why am I opening up to you about this? Well, to be honest I was not going to. I couldn't do it. But you see, through the course of my work, people have opened up to me about many issues, even this. Many have revealed how they've lost the drive to be intimate with their partner; they are in their head and can't enjoy the moment; they have lost their libido. People have revealed the most intimate and personal details to me, yet, still I hid in fear. But having thought it through, I am heeding my own advice: Talking does help. I felt it was only right for me – and for you – that I open up about this most heartfelt of struggles.

All those people who felt safe confiding in me have inspired me to be more open about this. My mental health problems fed my performance problems in the bedroom, and eventually my performance problems fed my mental health problems. It was a vicious cycle.

This may be happening to you. You want so much to be connected to your partner – or a partner. You want to ask that guy or girl out, but you're frozen with fear, and know there's no point in doing so because you're inadequate. This may happen to you in the future. Do you know what? It probably happens to us all at some stage. What I do know is that it's treatable, as with most things. Talking about the issue with your partner first and foremost, is key. Then talking with a doctor, a counsellor or coach will further benefit you, help you work through underlying issues that may be a contributing factor.

I had to find the source of my problems, and as with all issues and fears in my life, it was down to a fear of failing, a fear of not being good enough. These thoughts put me under severe pressure. I became anxious, leaving my partner confused, without explanation, before entering a world of darkness, myself. I now know that when I'm comfortable with my partner and we have a good connection, the chances are, things will go well. Yes, I'm still in my head at times, but now I'm more open; I breathe, give myself a chance, and try again.

So, don't hide it. This is another thing we can work through. Be open to the beauty of an intimate, loving relationship.

Neil's Notes

If you're in a relationship that's not working for you, then talk to someone, maybe a counsellor. Talk it out, sound it out first, maybe that's all you need. I would then recommend talking to your partner about how you feel. Be open and honest, because, as I said, they might be feeling the exact same thing. Don't let it go on without addressing it, or wait till the kids have reached the age of eighteen before you address it. By then you're older, more set in your ways and more likely to say, ah sure why change now!

Don't dwell, act now!

—◆—

Depression doesn't discriminate.

Pieta House is a counselling agency for suicidal depressives, amongst other things. I remember that first day I walked, hopelessly defeated, towards the main door, I lifted my head for a brief moment. As I did what I noticed will stay with me for the rest of my life. A young person accompanied by an adult, presumably a parent, passed me by. Then another. Teenagers.

It really struck a chord with me that people so young were here for the same reason I was. They, too, believed that life wasn't worth living. It shocked me. I couldn't believe someone so young could have such thoughts or problems so big to harness such thoughts. Like me, self-harming and contemplating suicide were the only options left open to them.

It hit home. It hurt me to see people so young feeling as I did. I was at least 20 years their senior. I had more life lived, and so the situation I was in it could be a little bit more understandable, but them? So young. Only starting out in life. The penny dropped. I was that teenager. The 15-year-old writing 'suicide' and 'I want to die' in his bulky science book one evening in his bedroom at home in Kerry.

When I think of those young people that day and others I've come across, I beam with pride. Those young people had the courage to speak out. They are there getting the help they need for one reason, and one reason only. They eventually opened up, and talked. The courage, the strength, the bravery and the ability for them to be able to talk inspires me to find my inner strength. My inspiration, through many a low patch, has been the thought of those amazing young people.

This strength to talk can come when you least expect it. Earlier on in the book I mentioned I was asked to give a talk to 16-year-old students in a school in Co. Cork. I never mentioned the event which happened the following day. I received an email from a student, let's call him Sean, who was in attendance.

Let me just take you back to the day of the event.

For Sean this was just another school day to struggle through, granted someone new was coming in to speak to his class. Little did he know that this day would be the one in which he garnered all the strength he didn't even know he had, and took action to seek help. Sean was in a bad way, not knowing what to do or where to turn. He contacted me. I was amazed. It really did catch me off-guard. This shows you that the power of sharing our story will pull on the strings of others and tempt them to do the same.

His email arrived, and I felt the urgency behind the words. I phoned him as soon as I could. It might not be proper protocol, but school was out for two weeks, and I felt I had no other option open to me. I had presented my talk on a Friday, which happened to be the last day of school term, before they would leave for Easter holidays. I did not see the email until early Sunday morning. That was an important factor when deciding to call Sean.

'I'm so proud of you,' I said – and it was true, because he had taken that incredibly difficult first step and opened up to me about his problems. I continued to tell him. 'I'm so proud of you because you're twenty-one years ahead of me.' As you now know it took me over twenty-one years to reveal my problems. But Sean had just done it, at age 16. He got it, the importance of telling someone.

As the call was coming to an end, he asked me to not tell anyone. But this was something I could not promise. I let him know that I would have to contact his teacher and he reluctantly agreed. Sean's teacher, Hughie, is a friend of mine, so we chatted and he took the next steps. Trying to contact the principal without success, he then decided to contact Sean's parents. He made contact with his mother. Sean's mother couldn't get her head around what Hughie was telling her. The mother was confused as her son was in the same room as her and seemed perfectly fine (The mask!).

Shortly afterwards, Sean phoned me and asked why his teacher had called his mom. He told me his parents didn't buy into it. They didn't see anything wrong with him. My next step was to find someone in close proximity to Sean. Someone who would understand. Luckily, his brother, a guy in his mid-twenties, got on the phone. He was a calm and a rational thinker, who had some experience of this situation as he'd supported some friends going through similar things. He was a Godsend. He chatted to his parents, knowing they did not understand, but he kept them informed. He then took his brother for food and a chat. Sean felt much better by being able to open up and the fact his brother was there for him on a continuous basis.

Sometime later (two years) a thank you card was received from Sean, who was now in college, much happier, much freer and now excited about what the future held for him. If I had not been brought in by my friend, Hughie, to speak to his students that Friday, who knows what might have happened. Not only did Sean live to tell the tale but one of his best friends called me a couple of days after my first phone chat with Sean. He, too, was struggling and needed help, and help he got.

Those teenagers in Pieta House that day were also twenty-one years ahead of me. They had opened up and gave themselves the best chance to live a better life. If I were able to snap my fingers and all masks dropped to the floor, you would be shocked to discover how many have been hiding behind them; exactly like the one I wore for two decades.

When I released my blog and put myself and my mental health problems out there into the world, I received many messages from people opening up to me. Messages from people I had known in my youth, whom I would never for a second have thought suffered. They had no idea I, too, had struggled. I had messages from acquaintances, from friends of friends, from readers of my articles. They were so varied and so touching. I believe there are more people masking what is happening within. You might be one of them. If so, I urge them, and I urge you to become one of those we do know about – be the one who talks. Lower the mask.

Because so many of us wear this mask, it has led me to respectfully disagree with the previously stated statistics that one in four/five people will suffer from a mental health problem. Why you might ask? Well, I disagree with this statistic because I could never have been included in any statistics. How could I? Nobody knew about me. It was only when I opened up and went to Pieta House that I became a statistic. And this would be similar for those of you who contacted me, and by so doing opened up for the very first time.

I will say this again and again, so sorry if it irritates you. I want you to know, you are NOT alone. You are not alone in feeling the way you do; alone, sad, exhausted, not normal, wanting to die. There are so many of us out there who will relate to you and your problems. I want you to take the step and *become a statistic*. Open up about your problems and take action by getting the help and support you need. Being a statistic has saved my life!

Why am I stuck here?

It probably has become apparent to you now as to why I was stuck in this state. Having falsely believed I had tried everything I could, to change and help myself. I felt there was no more that could be done; falsely believed, as I did not try everything. Yet I still believed it was time to give up and end this misery of a life I lived.

By now you know I questioned this false belief. I did not try everything to stay afloat in this life. I wasn't in the right mind to. Trying something would have been extremely difficult and risky for my fragile state. I was masking. So that alone was blocking me from trying new ways to manage my mental health problems. If I did happen to try new action steps, then I wasn't consistent with them, growing impatient, wanting change to occur on demand.

This of course does not happen. You need to give it time. Be patient and keep learning. Why I was stuck for so long is down to many factors: Not accepting my situation; not really changing anything; not backing myself and believing I could change my situation; and not taking any action.

Chapter 8
Just talk will ya!

There are many advertisements from professionals telling you to do this and that, get the help you need, all you have to do is ask. Well, if asking was easy, then we would all do it, right? I was behind a mask, blocked and giving up. I'm often asked why I didn't tell someone about what I was going through. I mean, hell, if I'd known it was so easy, sure I'd have talked until the cows came home!

If only it was that easy. Unfortunately talking is not all that easy. Well, for some of us anyway. Would you agree? In fact, it's bloody hard, and no matter how many times you have talked before, it can always be quite daunting. What people need to realise is that you're talking about something maybe for the very first time. You will be revealing something which you've gone to great lengths to hide, and which is so personal and so private. On top of that it's something you don't fully understand, yourself. So, you're expected to communicate these feelings and express this pain in words, to someone who might not have a clue as to what you're talking about.

Sometimes there is no rhyme or reason at all as to the depressive episode or bout of anxiety you experience. So how do we explain that one? And remember, this talking could be a first time for you or the person you're opening up to and so it needs to be a good experience in order for you to be able to do it again.

Throw into the equation that you're fearful of being judged by the people you tell. They might not mean to judge but you can see it in their expression as you pour your heart out. They are unwittingly judging, because they don't understand what you're going through. They might even at times question as to how the hell you could be low about something they see as trivial.

But remember, they are not you. You are not them. We all experience and feel things differently.

I began to fill my head with thoughts like: What if talking doesn't work; what if I feel no change? Then I'm really fecked, right? Talking and opening up needs to be a continuous process and not a once-off. That is very important to understand. It can be difficult to believe that the talking process is working, leading us, instead, to gravitate towards thoughts of the fallout of a failed process. This is a very real concern.

When I talked and opened up for the first time, I had myself convinced that I had played my one and only 'get out of jail' card. I felt I could not do it again. I could not bother someone again and again and again with my 'nonsense' right? Well thanks be to God I don't listen to myself all the time! I've learned, since then, that *you have to* talk again and again and again. There is no limit to talking. It should be this continuous process which is done whenever you need to. No limits put on it.

Don't fall into the trap I did of over-thinking it. Just do it. Do not *only* talk about your feelings when they hit, but also talk about past experiences, what you went through, talk it all out. This is what talking and opening up is all about; leave nothing behind, and make the most of this newfound relief.

Talk NOW, and Talk OFTEN.

Unfortunately, there are people who, for many reasons, will never come out from behind their mask. Nothing will move them to do it. Maybe that's you. Well, that's okay. Of course, I would love you to talk. But if that's too much then I understand. But what you have to do is, you still have to do something. Try some form of meditation. Try writing your thoughts down. Try adopting my or others' advice, and making it your own. Whatever that something is, doesn't matter, but please do something and explore what can work for you. Please, promise me!

The fear is real!

Fear, for me, had many faces when going through depression or anxiety, and when I had those suicidal thoughts. It's not a light-hearted topic of conversation. Not the easiest topic to find ways to kickstart a chat in, 'Ah, yeah when I opened my eyes this morning, I wanted to die, sure, you know how it is, yeah?' It's a topic which could potentially have an adverse effect on some people, to the point that they might feel somewhat afraid or uneasy around me. The last thing I, or you, need is for someone to react in a way which increases this fear of speaking out.

People have to understand that this topic, our mental health problems, is something we live with and try to deal with on a daily basis. That does not mean we understand it or can explain it. When you don't fully understand it yourself then it's hard to convey what you mean or feel to an outsider. With this lack of understanding, and an inability to communicate our problems, is the real fear that when you try your best to open up, the person you choose to speak to might react in a way that could do more harm to you than good. That person might judge you. They might try to hide it but they might distance themselves from you. They might have nothing more to do with you, and you will have lost more by opening up than by keeping quiet. This is the last thing you need on top of everything else. So why run the risk? Better to keep my mouth shut, and struggle on.

Fear of being noticed

I feared standing out from the crowd. If you knew me then you might question this because I really can be noticeable in a crowd. That attention seeker, full of chat and laughs and jokes. But that was my mask. That was me putting you off the scent of my all-consuming depression, anxiety and constant thoughts of suicide. I didn't want you to know about my problems because I did not want to stand out. I did not want for you to know I was different. I did not want for you to see me differently, even though I'm sure there might have been times when people have viewed me as a little strange. I would rather it be said that I'm strange than labelled for life as the guy with mental problems. It's strange, how things change. I just gave myself a quick google there. All the results bar none have mental health labelled to the headlines connected to my results. Anxiety, depression and suicidal ideation are all there associated with my name and very much a part of who I am.

Fear of no way out

I feared always being like this. I could see no end to my depression and anxiety. I could see no reprieve to this desire to end my life and finally have peace. I feared this was my reality. I had plucked the short straw and this is just how my life was meant to be. Can you imagine thinking that for the rest of your life you'll live in a darkness?

The ever-present uncertainty related to depression and anxiety is in itself anxiety-inducing. Not knowing when the darkness will strike; how deep it will be; how long it will last; how much strength and energy I will have to summon this time in order to battle through; whether I will be able to keep the mask up to the outside world; the uncertainty of how long a reprieve I will have until the next strike; and the uncertainty of knowing if I will be able to recover this time.

This fear is real. There is no way out. It will always be like this. So, what's the point in sharing this pain? It will be of no use whatsoever. These strong thoughts ensured that I remained stuck in limbo, blocking any hope of finding an alternative way out. And yes, there are alternative ways out, other ways to think about your mental health, other action steps for you to explore to help you move forward and through your own struggles.

Fear of being pitied

Do NOT feel sorry for me! It will do me more harm than good. I feared pity a lot. I don't want your pity. I don't want your approach to me to be any different than it was before. I don't want to be 'Poor Neil', nor do I want to be the talk of the town or the online community. Please stop noticing me! Acknowledge my journey and just go about your day.

Being noticed all the time with those sorrowful eyes would actually drive me bloody mad. Don't change how you were towards me before you found out. 'Hey, if you didn't like me before, there is no need for you to like me now.' I'm the same person as before you found out, so PLEASE treat me so.

You might think this kind of odd, right? I don't want to be noticed or pitied yet I've exposed my struggles and my personal story through newspaper articles, a documentary, radio stations, my blog, social media platforms and many talks at conferences and various companies. So, how the hell can I expect not to be pitied or to have sorrowful eyes feel my pain. Isn't the whole point of me telling my story so that you connect with me and feel that pain and suffering I went through. Yes, that is the point. I want you to connect but I want you to pass through the pity and sorrow and find the hope in my story. Find the strength and the want to stay alive. To help and support others to want to live this life. If we stay in the pity and sorrow then my story won't have the desired effect. But if we move through this pity and sorrow and use these emotions to drive our hope, then we can change lives; our own and others.

Fear of lost connections

I feared never meeting someone special. In 2014, the time I revealed my mental health problems, I was six years out of an eight-year relationship. I've had some interactions since, but nothing concrete. As I reflect back, a major reason for this was the narrative I had adopted. I had myself believe I wasn't ready or capable for a relationship at this present time (*this present time* being year after year after year). I had nothing to offer someone, so how could I be in a relationship when I didn't know myself, coupled with all those problems I had behind my mask? I wasn't ready to have this conversation with someone I wanted to have a relationship with.

On reflection, the longest term of any of these 'relationships' was three months, max. Even that was way too long for some of them to continue. But if I'm honest I was too weak and maybe too selfish to end them. Opting, instead, to wait it out until the other person ended it. And get this: Even though I knew the relationship should never have gone past maybe two dates, when the other person ended it, I felt like shit. It hit me hard. It took me a while to realise why: Because I was rejected again. Even though you could say that, in some way, I was the instigator, I still felt rejected.

It's okay, really, you can ask why would I do something to cause myself pain? Stay in a relationship which wasn't for me. It's a valid question and one which I have asked myself. I think the sad truth of it is that I wanted to have an outlet. Someone to connect with. To help take my mind off my reality.

Do you know, I can sit here today and say I don't need to have anyone in my life, and mean it? I'm much stronger now, both inside and out. Well able to live life alone. But why not live it with someone you care about? Why not share all those life experiences with a loved one? Yes, I would like to find that special someone, and enjoy the next phase of my life with them. Wouldn't you?

I totally believed that if I'd found the strength to reveal my mental health issues, then women would steer clear of me. Why the hell would they want to take on my problems? It's hard enough to just find someone without complications, never mind them having to deal with the uncertainty of my depression and all that goes with it. So, I truly believed that if I revealed all, then I could kiss goodbye any chance of a relationship.

But the truth is this: If a person doesn't accept you for who you are, warts and all, if you have to act differently around someone, then is this really the right person for you? Do they really care about you? Is the relationship doing you more harm than good? Remember, be true to yourself.

I do want to quickly point out that since being open and honest about my mental health problems, my experiences have been totally different. Most women I've met have been great, and I seem to have connected with them on a deeper level; some even having had a similar journey. I'm sure there are some who have thought, 'Not a hope, I'll steer clear of him,' and that's okay, too. I have to accept that some individuals won't want to get involved, and that's their right.

I'm glad to say, I don't regret, for one second, my decision to share my experiences. I've hidden behind many masks for way too long. It hindered me from being able to live a full life. Now, for the first time in over 21 years, I can say, 'This is who I am. I know I will meet that special someone one day!'

Fear of losing out

There is also the fear of revealing something personal, and still not being fully understood, or even accepted in society. Could it affect my job prospects or hamper my career progression? These, unfortunately, are very real fears which many of us carry.

And get this: I also thought that if I opened up to all, then my brother and sister-in-law would not allow me to look after my nieces and nephews. Friends wouldn't want me around their families, because who knows how I might act? In my head I hear them say, 'He could be depressed now, no, don't invite him over.'

Fear of being seen as a fraud

I feared that people would see me as weak, and question what I had to be depressed about. I think many of us question ourselves and our depression. I know I did. 'Jeez Neil, what the hell have you to be depressed or anxious about? You're not homeless, you're not fighting cancer, you haven't lost a loved one. You're a fraud. Nothing like this has happened to you. So why the hell are you feeling this way?'

These are real thoughts and questions you might be asking yourself right now. What I've learned, and now acknowledge, is that we're all different. We feel and experience things differently. Various traumas in my life went undealt-with, while a severe pressure and darkness was continuously building, with no release valve. This led to my major problems. I can't belittle them. They affected me. They are real. They are valid.

Fear of losing those close

I feared losing people in my life, be it friends, colleagues or family; similar to what's discussed above. Imagine losing those who are an important part of your daily life. It would be devastating. But, at the end of the day, it might sometimes be necessary. As we pass through the seasons of life, our circle of friends changes. People move in different paths. If people move away from you when you reveal something like this, then they are not the friend you want. I know you might say, 'Oh, it's easy for you to say.' No, it's not. I still crave friendships, but I now put the focus on me and how the friendship makes me feel rather than bending over backwards to please others.

Know this, you and your health are more important than what people think. People will think a certain way about you because they're unsure about themselves. They're uncomfortable in facing their own fears or addressing their own problems. I've learned to back myself, to do what is right for me, and not dwell on what others might think. It saved my life after all! Are you ready to put your health first, over what others might or might not think?

Chapter 9
Stigma

I know it's a lot harder than just saying, 'Yes, I will.' Yes, I will put myself first, and talk. For sure I will. The reality is, our state of mind, combined with the mental blocks we've built up, and the narrative our mind spouts each and every day, make it seem an impossible step to take.

This impossibility is intensified by the enormous role stigma plays in my silence. Only now, as I reflect back over my journey, can I grasp the role stigma played, though I did not really understand the root cause for remaining hidden behind my mask. I didn't name the obstacles which stood between me and escaping my struggles. If I had been able to identify and label these obstacles, then maybe I could have tried earlier to overcome them. Doing so could have helped unravel me from my pain. If we can't put our finger on the issues, then it's far more difficult to challenge and change them.

In the last number of years, I've really come to understand stigma. Through this understanding, I can now see the role it played in my silence. I can see the role or the hold it can still have on me to this day. One thing I now know for sure is that it had a major impact on my life, all through my life. I'm pretty sure that it impacts your life too. It impacts the vast majority of us who struggle day to day. So, are you open to learning a little more about stigma and its origins?

Stigma is a Greek word, which means 'the branding or tattooing of animals or slaves'. I'm sure we have all seen this on TV or in films, right? Animals being marked with a hot branding iron and, in some films and TV, people are branded as a form of torture. Not a nice vision eh! Also, did you know in World War II it was used to emblazon yellow badges on the jackets of Jewish people, in order to make them easily identifiable? They will stand out from the crowd and the rest of us will know that they are different from us. They were being labelled.

Next, you have to take a look at illnesses in the past. Leprosy was stigmatised. As was AIDS. So, stigma was a form of torture. It was used to highlight the fact that you were different. It was used to demonstrate that you should be avoided, that you're the lowest of the low, that you should not be treated in the same way as other humans.

And now you want me to talk about my mental health problems? Are ya havin' a laugh? You think I'm going to allow myself to be labelled like that? Do you think I'm going to allow myself go through a similar but more modern-day torture and ridicule? Now, there's a stigma around mental health. It's people with mental health problems who are labelled and branded. So, not a hope in hell! I will keep my mouth shut, thank you very much. Come to think of it, this mask, yeah, mmm, it fits me pretty good, yeah I... I actually like it, the comfort you know! Think I'll keep it on. It suits me! Conversation closed!

Am I the only one who thought this way? Are you thinking the same? Are you thinking it's just a better choice to stay behind the mask and suffer in silence?

This fear is real, right? As I mentioned before, this fear of being labelled or people changing the way they see me, it was real. And yes, I can hear people's voices in my mind's ear, saying that this would not happen, that I would not be viewed differently. No, you don't think so? Well, I beg to differ, let's see if I can change your perspective.

Okay, I've got it. If I was in prison at one time and you were describing me to someone, how would you do it? Would you say, you know the guy, he is bald, he is from Kerry, blue eyes. He has the most amazing smile ever, of course, like. Would the fact I was in prison *not* be mentioned? More than likely, it would, right? Do you think that label would stay with me for as long as I live, or do you think that after a number of years it wouldn't feature in my description anymore?

Sorry, but even a few months would be too long for it to follow me around. It could be detrimental to my health. Do you think I would put this fact about me on a CV for a job? Would people not look at me differently if I'd been in prison? Still not convinced? Okay, that's fine.

Let's look at another quick example.

Take AIDS. If I had AIDS, would you say, 'He is the guy who has AIDS'? Would you be a little more wary of being around me? Would you drink from the same cup as me or eat from the same plate? We have all seen the movies and fear in people's eyes when confronted with someone living with AIDS. To be honest, when younger I would have thought twice about being in someone's company who has AIDS. Luckily today we are more informed about it, but it is still surrounded by stigma and discrimination. I remember catching myself thinking when I heard someone had AIDS, I thought, 'Oh I would be careful there'. We all do it. So, I know for a fact (yes, a fact) that others will label me and be wary of me when they find out. So again, NO THANK YOU! My lips are sealed.

Note: Above I mentioned AIDS and that at one point in my life I would have been wary of people living with AIDS. The reason was because I wasn't informed around it. Now, I'm better informed, so would not have the same viewpoint. That, for me, is the key. I became informed and so less wary or if I'm honest, less afraid. Becoming fully informed about a condition, like our mental health, will help in the fight against stigma. That means you and I can play a massive role here. We can share our stories, give mental health problems a much-needed face and help people to become more informed and receptive to mental health conditions. How cool is that?!

As we have seen, stigma is not unique to mental health problems but it is rampant in society in relation to depression, anxiety and suicidal ideation. For me, there are two types of stigma. My friend Rob Cronin, a counsellor from my home town in Killarney, labels them 'public stigma' and 'self-stigma'. I refer to them as external and internal stigma. Whichever one you decide feels right, it doesn't matter, what matters is we have to contend with both types, not just one. This creates an even greater challenge for us to overcome in our push to talk about it.

External stigma is what I've just been talking about. If I reveal to you that I'm suffering, I'm open to your judgement. I believe this reveal indicates that I have a lack of opportunities open to me, in career, in love, in friendship, and in life in general. I will be viewed as weak, excluded from events and activities. Well, you get it, the list goes on! All in all, I will stand out like a sore thumb, and be labelled by you and everyone else. Simple as!

The internal stigma really came to light for me after I made my pain known. I realised that I was the cause of some of this stigma. You might be asking how I came to this conclusion. If you recall, I was saying I had this fear about opening up and talking. I mentioned that this fear was real for a number of reasons: Fear of losing people, being noticed, and being seen as weak. But these are all internal fears, right? They have no real basis; how could they? Because I, (at the time) had never put them to the test. I might have heard stories about other people's experiences when they shared their pain, but I, Neil, had never put these fears to the test. So, how can I make such claims? How could I know that this will be the case? How could I know that the people I tell will have this reaction? I couldn't!

Therefore, I'm envisaging the reactions people will have, before I give them a chance to actually react. I'm running with a narrative that has no foundation whatsoever, regarding me, personally. In effect, I'm labelling everyone with the same brush, which is not fair. I'm doing unto others, that which I do not want done unto me.

I know I should not do this. It's not fair to those people around me, to those who would be there for me in my time of need. Even when people won't understand what I'm going through, many of them will step up and be of immense support.

You need to eradicate the belief that others will judge you and look at you as an outcast. Give people the benefit of the doubt. Give them a chance to help. Yes, some might react in a negative way but I can guarantee that the vast majority will react in a very positive and supportive manner. The beauty about this is that you have the power within you to address this internal stigma. Give it a try!

Chapter 10
Is suicide the only path?

As the tough times took their toll on me, mentally and physically, without any relief, the idea of suicide became a more tangible idea. It then became a want as well as a need. A want, because no end was in sight to my never-ending suffering. A need because I was just so exhausted. This constant battle, constant struggle, the battering and my day-to-day pretence was getting the better of me. Which I think is clearly evident from my first words in this book - *'time to close my eyes to the world'*. The want to die was just so great. For me, following the light was to die and this is the only way I would ever have the peace I needed. I was exhausted. I needed to go. I want you to realise that the decision to die, again this is from my own experience, is not one taken lightly. It's seen as the only remaining option. One which, in the long term, will benefit me, my family and friends. As my pain and suffering grew so too did this belief.

People close to me have taken their lives; I've seen first-hand the impact and tragedy it has left behind.

A friend

Shane died over eight years ago. He was in his thirties. Shane was, as they say, tall, dark and handsome, and yes, a girl magnet. He was intelligent. I mean REALLY intelligent. I can remember when we were in maybe 3rd year in secondary school in St. Brendan's college Killarney. We were in the middle of honours maths class (I lasted a few weeks before being kicked out, haha). As the teacher went through a new type of maths problem, I looked to my right and Shane wasn't writing and had no copybook. I can still see him very clearly sitting at the desk. I was thinking, what the hell? I'll never forget it, he was sitting there, paying attention, nibbling on the sleeve of his jumper, and taking it all in. Shane would ace those exams and never have to put in as much work as the rest of us. That was the level of Shane's intelligence. He went on to become a designer working in Dublin, then moving on to the UK. While in the UK Shane changed profession and started working with animals. He also had some story about meeting, or getting to know an extroverted TV personality and fashion critic. But that was Shane, always finding himself in some outrageous situations with a good story to tell.

When I received the news that Shane had taken his own life, it triggered memories right back to our childhood, when we used to play outside in our estate; football (soccer) being one of our favourite pastimes. Shane was often the goalie and I remember that his attire was the Packie Bonner's yellow Irish goalkeeper jersey, with a pair of Levi jeans. If you grew up in the 80's you know Levi's were the real deal and usually worn for special occasions rather than being subjected to the mud, sweat and tears of one of our tensely fought football games. But Shane was Shane, having not a care in the world – or so we thought.

Memories play an important role in our lives, and surface when triggered by current events. These memories are from moments you've had in the past, and more than likely moments which you've shared with the people you care about. My message to you is: Create moments. As many as you can, because those moments will become memories which you'll cherish for a lifetime. I'm glad I created some special moments with my childhood friends, including Shane. As I now have those memories to keep me going, especially when the hard times hit.

I remember one meeting we had, when Shane had arrived back in Dublin for a few days from London. We met for a few pints in the then Russell's pub in Ranelagh, in Dublin, and chatted. He was sharing stories about his work with animals and, of course, the beautiful women he'd met (not jealous, I swear). Sharing his plans for his mother's house in South Kerry. He was a designer, and had plans for the interior decor of the house, and was sharing how he was ready to move back to Ireland, having secured a job. All seemed to be going well for him. Exciting projects and moves on the horizon. I was happy for him even though I, myself, was struggling.

I was lucky enough to have another one-on-one chat with Shane at our friend Paul's wedding in Kerry. We went to an outside bar and shot the breeze for a while about childhood and future plans. Again, his future looked so bright. There are some people in life, you don't see often but when you do, there's no work to it, everything flows so naturally. Shane and my childhood friends are those people. There's no work to it, you can be you. Well, you know what I mean!

I often think back to the night in the pub in Dublin and think how similar our lives were in some ways. We were both moving locations to, I suppose, find something better. We were both not-settled, both single; maybe because we were not settled inside ourselves. Looking back on it, I think we were both lost. I know I wasn't thinking that Shane could be lost in the same sense that I was. How wrong was I? I ask myself why didn't I connect the dots. Why couldn't I see him? Could I not see the signs in how his life was going, because as I said our paths seemed similar?

Unfortunately, I think the answer is something I'm very familiar with. It's the same reason nobody noticed me. We mask it; we hide it very well. The mask rarely drops in front of people. If I'm right, then Shane wore his mask well, just as I did! I was probably too consumed in my own darkness and my own masking of my problems, too worried about letting my own mask slip (It does take a lot of energy, you know!).

The funeral had his friends, old and new, in attendance, including us childhood friends. Funerals are strange experiences; you go through an array of emotions under a black cloud. It's a touching and reflective day, one where stories are shared, giggles had, and tears shed. At one time, I found myself stopping and taking everything in, noticing the pain his family and friends were going through. I too, like others, was confused as to why he did what he did, even though I knew his pain (from my own experiences) all too well, and maybe even his reasons. Was it the same want for a relief as I had? Did he, too, believe he'd tried everything humanly possible to help himself, and come to the realisation that things would never change, leaving him with only one option? Even though, at the funeral, I was seeing and feeling all this pain, I was, believe it or not, actually jealous. I was jealous that Shane was free, and I was still having to deal with my shit. When I think about it now, it does sound crazy, that after the shock, the confusion and the pain, jealousy was beginning to consume me. I was jealous of someone who was no longer living.

Funerals and death are a part of life, but that doesn't make it any easier. What I hate about funerals – and there is a lot to hate – the one thing I find really hard is, once they are done, time moves on.

It's true we grow stronger with time, or maybe we can just deal with the pain a little better, but for me as time goes by it, too, means more time living without the person who died. Years have passed since Shane. Still so hard to believe and understand but I'm thankful I've got those beautiful memories to warm me during the most difficult of moments.

If only they had told us!

A question I try to answer, when I speak at events or workshops, is one that all family and friends impacted by suicide ask: Why? Why didn't they just talk to us? As I have already mentioned, when people are struggling with depression, the decision to keep quiet isn't black and white. You just want the pain to stop because the fight is exhausting. The draw of death is too good to pass up. The relief it will give is much needed. I'm sorry, but in the end, it's as simple as that. If the person did at one time open up, but still took their own life, they might have, as I know I did, come to believe that it wasn't working. Because they were still suffering, and there definitely was no other way to end it. You become so exhausted, so tired of being dragged through barbed wire that you can no longer do it, no matter the pain and suffering left behind. The desire to stop battling, and to just have peace, is so great; and yes, we know the pain and hurt we will cause. But we feel that in the long term it will cause much less pain and hurt to all of those around us.

Think about my feeling of jealousy towards Shane. Even though I saw and felt the total impact it was having, and would continue to have, on his family, I still wanted to die. That should tell you everything. It's not a selfish act, even though I understand why people might think and feel it is. It's the only act we truly believe we have left.

I used writing as a tool to help myself and try to get these thoughts out of my head. The following is a thought I had written in the aftermath of Shane's funeral. Eleven days after, to be exact:

…it's inevitable, …death, …No, not from old age, …Self-inflicted; overdose, hanging, jumping, or crashing.

Even after I talked about my problems, I still harboured feelings of suicide. About two weeks after I revealed my mental health problems, I remember my brother asking if I was okay. I think he must have noticed a dip in my form but I gave the good old Irish reply, 'Yeah, of course, I'm *grand* sure'. But I wasn't; I was in a bad way. I was struggling big time again. Even though I had already talked about my problems, and was open, I couldn't force myself to do it again.

I'm repeating myself; I know. But it's important. I felt that by opening up already, I had used up my get-out-of-jail-free card, and so I felt I couldn't bother anyone again with my negativity. I knew people would be sick of listening to me go on and on and on about my problems. I know what you're thinking, it makes no sense whatsoever, but to me it made perfect sense.

If you're struggling and feeling this way then listen to me now. Open up, *always* open up. Let me put it to you this way: What would your family rather you did? I asked myself, would my family rather have me speak over and over and over again about my negative experience (as I so wrongly labelled it), and they have to listen, or would they rather that I never talk about it again, but seek another solution to help myself, being suicide, and in doing so taking away any chance they (my family and friends) would ever have to help me?

So, which option do you think your family and friends would choose? Would they want to have that choice? Rather than you take it away from them. You and I both know they deserve that chance!

I just wish I could turn back the hands of time, and know then what I know now, and be able to help those I truly care about. I know now that I didn't have to be alone, or endure this loneliness; none of us do. And you don't, either. As you read this you might think it easy for me to say, but it's not, I still, at times fall back into some darkness, but now the difference is, it's not so dark, it's not dark for as long as it used to be, and not as often. People are there for you, just give them the chance. They deserve it, don't they? I'm here for you, and these are not just words. You can contact me and I will be there to connect, and you'll learn eventually to win from within.

Even though I wish so much that I could turn back the hands of time, I'm not so sure things would be different. We ask ourselves why we didn't see what was happening, or notice anything out of the ordinary, but turning back time, and being in that situation again doesn't mean we would notice. This *noticing* is a message I've been very vocal about for years. That if we were just to *notice* someone, then we could save them, and maybe ourselves, a lot of pain and suffering.

If you and I could notice someone when they are suffering, then that would be unbelievably life-changing. But noticing can be so hard to do, especially when you get someone like me, who has mastered the art of wearing a mask. If I don't want you to know, then you won't know. I can guarantee that, and my twenty-one years of masking is testament to that fact.

In 2014, when I spoke out, many people commented on some posts and articles I wrote. A friend from Killarney, Brian Parker, in 2014, wrote this message underneath one such article: 'I have known Neil well for about 8-9 years, and lived with him for one of those years. I would never have known (or as he would say, *noticed*) that Neil was suffering in the way he was and is. When he told me, one night earlier this year what was really going on in his life, I was shocked and surprised, to say the least, mostly because at any stage in my life when times were tough, Neil was one of the first people I would have talked to. He still is. Never one to turn away from a challenge, I'm hopeful that the road Neil is now on will open people's eyes and minds to *noticing* the issues people face. As Neil says it's the noticing which is difficult and I can vouch for that.'

This was one of the many amazing messages from my friends. This one stayed with me because it really shows how convincing my mask was. As Brian said we were even housemates for a year and he never witnessed what I was going through and, as you now know, my lows were so low and dark, and my anxiety was so extreme, yet he did not notice, and that wasn't down to him, but down to my skill of hiding it. Brian also goes on to mention that I was one of the first people he would have talked to about his problems. This is so true, and I can say it's true of many of my friends. I would listen to their problems and offer support, advice and guidance through their tough times. Something, it seems, that I was quite good at, which is bloody ironic, right? I could do none of this for myself, or so I had myself believe. I also think that focusing on others and their problems is a great distraction from our own. It allowed me not to have to focus internally and deal with my own demons. It's always easier to help deal with someone else's, even as we are slowly dying inside.

Hello! Are you still there?

Well, how are you doing now? Are you still with me? I hope you're doing okay, and if you feel the book becoming too much, then stop. Put it down and do something you enjoy, preferably in the fresh air.

In the next section we are going to look at 'The Path' I forged for myself, by leaning on all my experiences. So hopefully a little bit of a lighter read but, again, I do appreciate you joining me on this journey and I hope you're able to identify with and now see hope in relation to your situation.

Before I move on to the next section do you mind if I ask you a question or two?

How do you feel about me right now?

After all you have read, how do you feel about me?

Do you feel sorry for me?

Am I weak to you?

Sit with the questions for a bit, and answer them honestly!

Okay, I'm going to have a shot in the dark here: You feel that I'm brave, you feel sorry for me, but don't think I'm weak? Am I right or anywhere close?

Well, in a way, yeah, I do believe I'm brave, in having dealt with all that I have; but my bravest step, I think, is one you have yet to read about. By now you know I don't want you to feel sorry for me. Empathy to a degree, yes, but not pity. You being sorry for me doesn't help me. It actually makes me feel less, if that makes any sense.

Last of all I know you don't think I'm weak; well, hopefully not anyway. You are right, I am not. Having to deal with this shit I go through and to come through it and move forward in my life is one of the greatest shows of strength I have ever made. So, I'm not weak; I'm fucking strong, even if I do say so myself. Well, my friend, so are you. You're just as strong, if not stronger.

So now, use this strength to continue reading this narrative of my journey, whilst at the same time stepping forward yourself. See you on the next page 😊

PART TWO

The Path

Chapter 11
Time to change

You have no idea how difficult and exhausting it is for me to be out in public and, in fact, how hard it is at times to sit and write this book. The book has taken me longer than I hoped, mainly due to revisiting such personal details. When I write about such experiences, I'm in it, I feel it. At times I have to stop, walk away and collect myself. This, believe it or not, is good; it's progress. I now know when I need to stop, take a break, and change my scenery. This wasn't the case before I talked, and discovered that I had to make a decision once and for all.

So, decision time!

'To be or not to be, that is the question'. Such indecision, Hamlet, old boy! Unlike you, Hamlet, I've made my decision. I'm going to take my life. The time is now!

I had learned from personal experience that the uncertainty of indecisiveness creates unbearable anxiety, so I should just make a decision and feel that sweet relief. And boy did I feel good deciding to die. I had a future! It was a relief to know that I would no longer have to battle each day.

…….. As you can probably tell, I'm still here. Therefore, obviously, I did not go through with it. I hear your question. Don't worry, I've heard the same question many times now:

'Why did you decide not to take your life?

'What changed your mind?'

'How did you know you really wanted to live?'

I'm always happy to answer questions. So please keep asking, because learning from the experiences of others is, for me, the best way to become more aware and informed about mental health problems and the lives people with them live. We need to learn from each other. Please share. The telling of your story won't only help you but many others struggling on their own.

So, why didn't I kill myself? The short answer is: I don't really know. As far as I was concerned, I had tried everything to beat this depression but there wasn't anything more I could do to help myself. After coming to this conclusion, it was obvious that living, for me, was a waste of time and energy; only in death could I truly be at peace and relieved of this darkness forever (you'd swear I had insider information about what happens to us when we die!).

With my decision made, my focus turned to 'when'. When is a 'good' time to kill myself? Now that I reread that line, it's so surreal, what a bloody question to ask myself! I can actually feel the anger building within me as I write this. There is never a good fucking time to do it.

No second chances

Some of the following description is raw and might be triggering, so read to the end, and don't take this as permission to act.

With that said, if you're okay, let's carry on!

I firmly believe that many of those who have taken their own life would have been grateful for a second chance. If something had gone wrong during the act, say the rope snapped when trying to hang themselves, they would be so grateful that their suicide attempt failed. Up to that moment when you step off the chair, it seems like the right decision. But once you feel the snap of that rope around your neck and the air being cut off, if you question that decision, it's too late. You will never breathe air or see loved ones again. NEVER!

A number of years back I remember reading in the *Irish Times* newspaper a report coming from my home county of Kerry. It stated 'a coroner made an emotional plea at the end of his court after all but one of the inquests into deaths in south Kerry were found to be suicide'. So, five out of the six deaths in front of him were suicide. The article described how one boy shook hands with everyone at a party and had later been found dead by his dad on the sitting room couch. Another told of how a father, with a trembling voice, described how he frantically went in search of his son only to find him missing from his bed. 'I went to his best friend – no sign. I went to the wood – no sign. I went to his girlfriend's house – no sign.' The boy was eventually found by his uncle. I can't imagine what it must have felt like at that moment when the uncle found his nephew. I picture him trying to revive his nephew. Nothing. Him being powerless in his efforts. Would you ever get over it?

Those situations when you visit families who have recently experienced a loss is a very strange one. Not knowing what to say, wondering whether to speak to the family, questioning should you be there at all.

I remember the first time I was visiting a family where a member had taken their own life. Nothing can prepare you for this. Being greeted by the father. The shock he was experiencing was evident straight away; him not knowing what to say, but thanking me for coming. An image which will stay with me forever. After some awkward interactions, mainly on the part of myself, we all went in for a cup of tea and to meet the rest of the family. Eventually, the house was beginning to fill with family and friends. A hub of silent activity.

I remember following that visit I chatted to a friend of mine whose uncle worked as a coroner for some time. I can remember him telling me that his uncle once said that he believes, as do I, that many of those who take their lives change their mind. That conversation with my friend that day is burned into my memory, but one detail stands out most poignantly: his uncle believes this because he has come across many bodies with scrape-marks on their neck from their nails.

How heart-breaking is that? Knowing your loved one wanted to stop it, to live. That must be soul destroying. If only they had talked to family, to someone, to anyone.

I won't apologise for repeating myself when I say: As difficult as it is, talking can save your life, and I was about to find out the true meaning of this.

The day that saved my life

On Monday 14th April 2014, a few weeks after I made the video, Time to Close my Eyes to the World, I allowed someone else to notice my suffering. That Tuesday morning, I called in to my sister-in-law, Sinead, for a chat. As I entered the house, the nutty aroma of brewing coffee filled the air. I entered the kitchen to bright rays of sunlight hitting the floor, counter and walls. The beautiful morning in all its splendour entered through the big glass double doors which led out to the garden, or, as I personally call it, my sanctuary. I stood there, as Sinead was making the coffee, recalling silent memories of having such fun with my nieces and nephews. On the trampoline, me being jumped on by four kids under seven years of age; playing basketball; or playing soccer into the well-worn goals.

With coffee in hand and chit-chatting with Sinead, about family, work, and all the rest, I suddenly had the realisation that I had gone off topic. I had started to talk about my situation, where my head was, where my life was going or, rather, not going. I wasn't holding back.

'I can't do this anymore,' I said. 'I can't go on. I just don't want to be here anymore. I want quiet. I want peace. I need rest.'

Sinead wasn't sure what I was talking about. 'Work?' she asked, maybe thinking work was getting on top of me.

'No, life,' I told her. She looked confused. 'I can't go on. I want to die.'

She is lost for words. Neil, the happy guy, the not-a-care-in-the-world guy, what on earth? I know I need to explain it in a way that she will be able to understand my pain, my suffering and my desire to die. I don't want to suffer anymore. I want to be free.

'You know how much the kids (my nieces and nephews) mean to me, how I would do anything for them? I love hanging out, spending time with them.'

They do mean the world to me. They've been my safety net, given me inner peace on the days when I've struggled. When with kids you can't but be present, in the moment. They demand all your attention. My nieces and nephews always demand uncle Neil (or King Neil as I would blackmail them with McDonald's to say) to be energetic, funny and always engaging with them. When I'm low, these features are the furthest thing from my mind and body. However, in their presence I couldn't but lose myself. At times when I was low, I would pay them a visit to escape my reality for just that brief period.

I continue, 'But even though this love is strong,' a rare smile appears when I think of the joy they bring our family, 'even though I want to protect them, as I do all my family, I know when I'm no more; this will never be possible again.'

'Even though my being gone means that life as my family know it will change forever, never again needing to call out my name, to share a secret, to wonder how my day is going, to be excited when I visit. Even though my actions will destroy my family as a whole; 'even though Saoirse (my eldest niece and my goddaughter) will have more birthdays, a 21st, become an adult, will never get to spend Neil and Saoirse time again, will never be able to call me, I have to go.

'Even though Caoimhe will never be able to invite me again to attend one of her gymnastic events, or use me as a human springboard when showing me her new, crazy gymnastics moves, I have to go.

'And Patrick, even though I know he won't get to spend days with me, just hang and shoot the breeze, or draw pictures for me anymore, I have to go. When I go to a soccer game of his, when he looks to the side line, I won't be there.

'And Liam, he won't be able to call me from the car after a game, to tell me he scored a goal, he won't be able to run to the front door when he hears the doorbell, and hug me. He'll never be able to watch a Liverpool FC game the same way again. Myself, Liam and my brother Paul would be sprawled on the couch in our usual positions, me on the right-hand side, Liam in the middle and Paul on the left-hand side, going through the emotional rollercoaster of supporting a team and celebrating when done. Even though I know he will never have this again, I have got to go!

'Even though…'

'I could go on forever about the hurt and loss it will cause. There are just so many. An endless list, but knowing all of this, knowing I will forever be an absent figure from everything family, I have got to go. The longing to be free, the want for peace, can only come with the ending of my life. This is all I want now. I want to leave this world behind; and yes, even when that means leaving you all; my family, the ones I love. I have to die!'

Holy shit!

I don't know how Sinead stayed so strong. I mean, it's the morning, you're chatting to family then – BANG! – the bombshell – **I can't go on**, I want to die. How is someone supposed to react to this? How are you supposed to provide support? How are you supposed to cope, yourself, when a family member tells you something you can never even contemplate; something that should never ever be part of our thought processes?

…but AGAIN I will tell you, I can guarantee THAT ANY FAMILY MEMBER, FRIEND, ACQUAINTANCE, COLLEAGUE, TEACHER, EVEN A PERSON ON THE STREET, would rather hear those unpleasant words from you than not hear them. They would rather deal with all the emotions flowing from those words rather than one day wake up and find you gone.

That morning was the first time I talked so openly about suicide. That day in April, the day I spoke out, is the day I allowed myself to be truly noticed.

It was the day that saved my life.

It was the day that changed my life.

I was lucky that I had someone like Sinead there, in that moment, on that day. Someone who was able to listen to something so shocking, and remain calm, which made me feel even more comfortable when revealing more of my hidden details. It was as if I was opening a 21-year-old pressure valve, which was close to exploding. If I had not had Sinead there that day, well then, I don't think you would be reading this book.

You've probably heard the expression: Not all heroes wear capes. This is what my family is to me. They are my heroes (even when they lounge around all day in their pj's). They have helped bring me back to life. I would do the same for them as they did for me, and as they continue to do on an ongoing basis.

Would you do this for your family or friends? I'm sure you would, right? Just as they would do it for you. One of life's great joys is being able to help someone. Did you know that you have the power to give someone the joy of being able to help you?

How do I help someone?

People often ask me, 'How can I help someone going through mental health problems?' or 'What do I do if they talk?' These are such valid questions and ones which Sinead must have faced so unexpectedly that Monday morning in April. I could see she was shocked, but she just listened and let me talk. Then she asked what could we do next? She didn't try to take charge of the situation or to issue instructions. That was the last thing I needed, and the last thing any of us need, in that situation.

Of course, there are going to be circumstances when you have to take the bull by the horns and do what you think is best for the person. This is something I personally experienced, not so long ago. This time I was on the other side of the fence: Noticing, listening and supporting. I and some others had to intervene and get much-needed help for a friend. Not an easy thing to do, but it was definitely in our friend's best interests. We had noticed changes in our friend's demeanour. He was acting out of sorts, and had become erratic. A few weeks earlier he'd confided in me about his past mental health problems, so this led me to become more aware of the changes occurring. Luckily, I wasn't the only one noticing and also showing concern. One Sunday morning, three of us voiced our concerns and decided to intervene, as our friend was rapidly declining.

We located him, and sat with him to explore what was going on. We didn't go in all guns blazing, ready to take control and make decisions for him. We had more of an exploratory and inclusive approach, and asking him what he felt was the first step. This is important as it allowed for him to buy into the process, ensuring that he would not distance himself from us. We could not afford for him to view us as being in opposition to him. We eventually, with the support of his family, got him the help he needed.

There are no set rules as to who we should talk to. More often than not, we just need an understanding ear, and that's what Sinead was for me. No judgement, no interrupting, just listening. It's important for the person to see that you're listening without being judgemental, that you're allowing the person to speak without interruption, because you don't want to give them a chance to rethink this decision to talk. If you want to clarify something with them, wait till you feel there is a pause and recount some point they made and ask if that's correct.

I never felt I would open up to anyone, let alone my family.

The family member will want to do the ultimate best, which can mean being very hands-on; instructing, directing, and taking the lead. Family members take the action THEY think is necessary, which might prevent them from truly listening. Of course, they want what is best for you, and think their course of action will serve you best, but sometimes their view is clouded by the proximity of your relationship.

This observation arrives from situations I've encountered, but it's not the same for everyone. People in a similar situation to me, might be more likely to open up to a friend or even a colleague, but each case is different. Do whatever you need to do in order to be heard, and if that means opening up to a family member then do it. There is no second guessing yourself. Remember, the most important thing is talk, so don't let the decision about who you should talk to be an obstacle.

There are no set rules on how to help someone. Guidelines, yes, but do whatever feels right in the moment. I helped another friend by sending a simple text. Simple for me, but an important support for my friend. Myself and this friend were open with each other about our mental health problems and I knew he could go into a deep depression every so often. I hadn't heard from him in a while so decided to call him for a chat. There was no answer, so I expected he'd call me back. A day or so passed and no call came. When I'm going through my dark spells, I won't answer calls, and I wondered if he felt the same. So I sent a simple message: *Hey buddy, I hope all is well. I'm here if you need anything, buzz any time. Chat soon.* I sent it, not expecting a reply. I knew it was important not to keep calling and texting, as this can put more pressure on an already dark situation. I also knew he was surrounded by family who understood his problems.

Two weeks passed before I received a reply: *Thanks man. Really appreciate the text. It kept me going. Thanks for the support.* How great was that? Even without me knowing it, my simple action of sending a text played a part in helping him through his tough time. The text reminded him that someone out there was thinking about him and ready to listen and support him in any way.

The power of something so simple can't be underestimated. A simple action for you and me could mean the world to someone else, and help them through, maybe, some dark struggle. We all want to be noticed to some degree, even if we think we don't.

Chapter 12
Is talking the answer?

It's okay not to be okay.

Thankfully this catchphrase has never been said to me. I wouldn't know whether to laugh or cry in frustration. This phrase has become popular on social media and is used by many organisations, activists, influencers and all those trying to raise awareness around mental health problems. It has also become closely linked to World Suicide Prevention Day.

I'm not a fan. It's not okay to be not okay.

I totally understand that people continuously repeat it, believing it will help those struggling feel less alone and for some it might do. For me, it had the opposite effect. I was suicidal and no, it's not fucking okay. I just want to *be* and *feel* okay. I'm sick of not being okay. I haven't been okay for over twenty-one years.

I think living within this statement can hamper our progress in dealing with our issues. I'd go as far as saying that this slogan could be used as an excuse to stay in victim mode. We might find some comfort in this 'poor me' zone, as it recognises that, yes, we have it tough in life and so should be afforded some leeway. This would, without any doubt, lessen the positive impact of talking and opening up, as we would then be talking for the wrong reason; for sympathy rather than support. Feeling sorry for a person does not benefit them in any way. It won't lead to a path towards sustainable good mental health. Talking is a tool that can empower, so let it be just that. And each time you talk, you'll gain in strength, confidence and belief.

That talking feeling!

I remember, so vividly, the feeling I experienced when I opened up to Sinead that day. I had heard that talking helps, but holy shit, this was amazing. I felt like running out into the street and shouting, *I'm cured, I'm fine now, woohoo*. The sense of relief I felt was fantastic. I tell you; it was as if someone had cut the puppet strings attached to me, which restricted my thoughts and movements, and I could finally stand on my own. I felt light and free. I smiled. A real and pure smile. If I had known relief was this instantaneous, I would have talked years ago. I felt so good in fact that I believed Sinead's job was done, and I was off to explore the outside world and my environment through my new lens.

Sinead is like, 'What? What do you mean you're off?'

'I've to go to the printing shop in Terenure', I said.

She tried to deter me, 'Ah, Neil, no; it might be better to stay here, you know...'

'Sinead, I feel great, seriously; thanks for that. I'm grand now, I feel great, thanks.'

Confused she said, 'Ah, no, look okay. Look, go do the job then come back, yeah?'

'Ah, okay, fair enough, I'll come back after,' I said. She stared at me. 'I promise,' I said. As I opened the door to leave, I shouted back to her in the kitchen, 'Oh Sinead, please don't tell Paul (my brother). I'm alright now, so, I just don't need any hassle.'

She barely nodded. I mean, was I for real? I was asking her to not tell her husband about such an important situation. I mean, Neil, wake up, man.

The honeymoon period

As I said, the relief of letting go of over 21 years of pain was immense. But I struggled to take this 'life changing' action again. It took me some time to realise I had to repeat this process constantly to help relieve my pain. When I talked, I immediately felt amazing, that is true. I would even say I felt on top of the world. The following few days I was walking on air, given a new lease of life. I had shed such a burden by opening up, and now, or so I would have myself believe, I wouldn't have to hide behind my mask anymore. Well, to my family at least. I could be myself. I mean, I could find out who I really was; what I liked, disliked, wanted to do with my life. There were endless opportunities for me to explore. I had left depression, anxiety and all those constant thoughts of suicide well and truly behind. Surely nothing could stop me now!

A few days later, this honeymoon period came crashing down. I did not expect this, sure why would I? I did what I had been told to do: I talked to someone. I opened up. I shared my pain. So, what was happening? On this car-crash of a day, I happened to meet my brother. He asked me how I was doing. I replied instinctively using the great old Irish expression, 'Sure, I'm grand'. But I wasn't grand. I was as bad as I had ever been. My depression and anxiety were once again kicking my arse and now my thoughts of suicide were even more compelling.

Paul must have noticed something because he asked me if I was sure, and I replied, laughing on the outside, and in turmoil on the inside, 'Yeah, sure, what'd be wrong with me'.

If you could have opened me up you would have found me at rock bottom, deep in my black hole, too exhausted and defeated to claw my way back out.

As my mood began to dip yet again, I began to think that this 'talking' was a total waste of time. How the hell is talking going to help me? I need more than talking, that's for sure. All these people on public forums telling people, 'Talk about your feelings', 'a problem shared is a problem halved'.

Oh, give me a break will ya! It did fuck all for me. I'm back where I bloody started. I talked. It didn't work, I opened up and it has done me no good whatsoever. Now I know for certain that I've tried *everything* possible. Sure, didn't I do what we are told to do? Didn't I? Didn't I talk as they preach for us to do and what, huh, what good has it done me? None! At least now I know there is absolutely nothing I can do in this life, in this body to help myself. I had lost.

Oh, shut up Neil! I can say this to myself, now I'm confident in being able to quieten the Neil of the past. Here he is spouting rubbish. Talking is NOT some magic wand you can wave and it will change everything. Talking won't erase my experiences of the last 21 years. It won't block the impending darkness or anxiety from attacking.

But what talking **will do** is help us to start the process of making sense of those past experiences. It will allow us to lighten the load. It will allow us to deal in a more positive way with those we have yet to face.

The 14th of April was a beautiful day; talking, releasing and escaping my problems, but it was a short reprieve, and once again, I shut myself off. What was worse was that I was being presented with opportunities from others to open up (my brother), and I didn't. I donned my mask once again and shut him and his support out. I needed him and his support more than ever, but I was closed off.

You might be saying to yourself, what the hell were you thinking? Why would you do that? Alright! Jeez all the questions! I've said, several times, that talking is hard, but most people don't tell you this. From my own experiences it didn't seem to get any easier; at least not in the beginning. You are revealing something so private and something which you don't truly fully understand. This in turn makes it difficult to articulate what you're going through, what your pain is and how it feels in your mind and body. And, of course, there's no logic to the low you're currently experiencing, so this makes it all the more difficult to discuss.

Add to this the fact that you're still fearful of being judged, that they just won't understand what you're going through. Others might view your triggers as something trivial and wonder how in hell someone could be low about something so basic. But you have to remember they are not you and you're not them; we all experience and feel things in our own unique way.

A final reason why I say talking is hard, and one which really played on my mind, was that I had told myself that I had already talked and revealed, and I did not want to put myself through that again. Nor did I want to be so selfish as to bother someone else over and again with my 'nonsense'. People have their own lives to deal with, they don't need me in their ear all the time. Is this true? Am I talking complete shite? How could you change your way of thinking?

Being able to open up and talk about your problems is an important tool to have in your arsenal. It took me a while to see it this way, but that's exactly what this process is; a continuous learning curve of trial, error, failure and success. You must be open to this, as each and every one of us will make some sort of mistakes in life. But as long as we learn from them, then mistakes become less significant and can propel you forward.

Neil's Notes

So, I learned to talk and talk and talk, and even talk some more. *You have to* talk again and again and again. There's no limit to talking. It should be a continuous process, a hard but much needed process. Don't fall into the trap I did, of overthinking it, just do it. Do not *only* talk about your feelings when they hit, but talk about past experiences, what you went through, talk it all out. This is what talking and opening up is all about, leave nothing behind, make the most of this new found relief.

Talking comes in many forms

Remember my video, mentioned on the first page of this book? Well, that's a form of talking, opening up and sharing my problems. A reason I found it very hard to speak out and open up was the fact that I had pictured myself sitting in front of someone, one to one. That thought and vision alone caused me great anxiety. It was another contributing factor for me keeping my mouth shut. Little did I know, there were other ways in which I could share these overbearing problems. Recording a video is one of many.

The end goal of talking about your mental health problems is to release all this built-up pressure and then for you to feel comfortable to continue to open up on a regular basis. I've learned to open up in many different ways, and each has its benefits.

If we look at my pathway to sharing my problems, it began with someone I trusted and felt comfortable speaking to. From there I reluctantly sought the help of a professional in the form of a counsellor. Did I know what I was doing in any of these situations? No, not at all. But a year or so after I opened up, I found myself an ambassador for mental health and well-being, speaking to audiences around Ireland. I've been doing this for some years now.

It's only now, writing this book, that I realise there are many beneficial ways for me to share my experiences, but also to help me in my daily process of managing my own mental health. Each time I open my mouth about my journey I relieve myself of a heaviness that could cloud my day.

You might not want to do talks or share your story on such a scale. You might not be ready to attend a counsellor but the point is, each time we express ourselves we release that build-up of pain. We prevent this bottling-up of emotions that need to be released. We are able to restore an order of more positive wellbeing, both physically and mentally.

You do whatever works for you.

Text someone, write down your feelings. Inform someone of what has been going on in your mind. This can be done also by email. The act of writing is super; something I still do. Getting that pain on paper or computer gives you a nice release. There are also counselling services via text or webchat, and phone lines to call and chat to a professional. If you look on any social media platform there are many moderated support groups where people can share their issues. These peer groups are not just limited to social media platforms, so use Google and find one for you. You could even do something like writing your thoughts in a journal, which I still do (I have a ton of writings from days when I was really low). You could record yourself on your phone (again which I have done). All of this helps, and is good practice for when you're ready to speak to someone else about your struggles.

Neil's Notes

Would you feel confident enough to try one of these many techniques, in order to help yourself? Which one do you think you might start with? Choose one and try it for two weeks. Then move onto another technique and keep building.

Go on, put down the book and try one right now!

—◆—

Chapter 13

Stepping onto a new path

The decision to take my life was not a major or conflicting one. I was at the point where it was the only option, and very much needed. Why would I want to move forward and live my remaining years like this? To die was the only option left to me, or so I thought.

I don't think I will ever succeed in describing the exhilaration I got from finding a new way to live. It's something I never thought possible in the slightest. I believed my time was done and my life would come to an end very soon.

Now, I'm moving forward every day. I've had many stops and starts on this new path and there have been countless times when I've wanted to give up, get back on that old shitty path and throw the towel in. This new path at times was so hard to deal with; it required so much energy and emotion to push on. Did I expect an easy ride? To prance through fields of flowers without a care in the world, like a Disney movie? Of course, it's going to be tough at times, really tough. There are also going to be beautiful moments that open up to you, which you might not see at first, but once the clouds of darkness lift, they become more obvious, more frequent and more sought after. The old path, the one I had lived for the majority of my life, does not even compare to this new one, even when, at times, I feel defeated while travelling it. I want more of this new path. I now know I'm worth fighting for and will do so forever more.

I found that I was beginning to ask myself if being on this new path meant I was over my mental health problems. I don't know. But what I do know, is that now I want to live. I am going to face these battles head on, as now I have the arsenal with which to deal with them. It's filled with tools I've explored and trialled and erred with, including meditation and exercise. It has recommended actions steps that I've adapted as my go-to actions, such as getting out into nature and adapting my day to meet my current need. These tools I can call upon to support and guide me through the battles.

I'm also ready to work at finding out how to avoid these battles. I'm ready to work at managing each battle and I'm ready to *not* think about when the next battle will be waged, and focus, instead, on the here and now. I'm ready for my new path in life and all the challenges and magical moments it will present to me. I believe in my self-worth, in my inner strength and my ability to adapt and progress. I continue to focus on where I want to go instead of being dragged back into my past life. Find hope in my words. Then take action to make your way onto your new path.

Eternal questions

Every time I struggled with an episode of depression, or was overcome with anxiety, I would ask myself the same questions time and again. Why me? Why the hell is this happening to me? And when is it going to end?

Is this striking a chord with you?

Do you find yourself asking similar questions?

Have you found the answers? If you have, then you are amazing. If not, don't worry because neither did I. I came to realise something even more liberating and progressive. Asking such questions as those above will do you no good. Focusing on them will stunt your progress, block you from moving forward with your life, and keep you firmly rooted in your misery and darkness, which has been your past. You need to not stay in a state of foreboding, but build your physical and mental strength on a continuous basis so that such questions become irrelevant and a part of your past.

In order for me to stop focusing on those questions, I had to turn my focus within, rather than on those 'happy' people all around who were living their 'happy' lives in their 'happy' world. It seemed everyone else had an understanding of life, and navigated it with ease, while I was left out of the big secret. It pissed me off that I was lost and confused. Why could I not just be like them? I just wanted what, seemingly, everyone else had, a simple life, a normal life. Was that too much to ask?

My tip is to stop asking 'why me!'

Why not you? Are we so special that we should expect an easy ride through life? Are we better than others? Do we deserve less struggle than other people? I don't think we do. And, as we've already established, not everyone has an easy ride through life, even if it looks like it. In fact, I would go as far as to say nobody does. We all have our crosses to bear, our pain to live with. So, STOP asking 'why me'. Just accept it, and move forward.

Also stop asking WHEN. When is it going to end? I said I will always be honest with you: I don't know. Nobody does. Has my darkness and anxiety ended? No, not at all. I get days where I struggle but, not to the extent as I once had. Nowadays, I can remain productive and active. Now I can even be out in public when I feel low or anxious, instead of locking myself away in my bedroom with the curtains closed, headphones on with the music blaring, so as not to hear the outside world.

I stopped asking 'when' a while ago. Now I honestly don't care. It could end tomorrow, in five days, in five months, in a year. It makes no odds to me. I move on regardless. That is the strength and confidence you get from accepting your situation, learning about you and accessing your power while building your own personal arsenal of resources, which will give you the strength to move on. You know what? My mental problems might never leave me, and if that's the case, well so be it. That is not my focus anymore. So, when are you going to start to focus?

You can do it, with loving support!

The beauty about this new path is, you don't have to walk it alone. The support I received on Monday, 14th April, 2014 did not just stop at listening. Even though I didn't want any more interference from people that day, I mean like, had I not done enough; spilling out my heart and head, warts and all? The support continued even though I might not have asked for it. You see we have to accept that there are times when we don't know what's best for us. Such times are when one needs to take on board the advice of others and listen to them for a change, rather than that voice inside our head. That internal voice has done us no favours whatsoever, has it?

If you can remember, I wrote earlier that as I left Sinead to do a job in Terenure, I asked her not to tell my brother what had happened, as I was now 'grand'? On my return to her house from Terenure, I rang the doorbell. They have this big black door which has a porthole sized window around head-height. I ring the doorbell and who comes out of the kitchen towards the door? YES! My brother, Paul! His jacket was still on, which told me he must have just arrived home. I started thinking, 'Ah shite, here we go, big brother instructing me to do this and that, he knows best, he'll lead the way, he'll be the action taker.' The door swings open. I step inside and wait for the instructions. Not a word is spoken. So here I stand in the doorway with my older brother, someone I look up to, as all younger brothers tend to do. I didn't want him to know. I didn't want to show weakness. I didn't want or need words of advice right now. I didn't want to be here. Why did I agree to come back to the house?

My worries were unfounded. I got no words, no advice, no instructions. What I did get is something I will never forget for the rest of my life: A hug! My brother just held me. No words just holding me. I don't know about you but I'm not used to hugs, especially from my brothers. I honestly can't remember if I cried but it certainly was the closest I'd ever come to crying in a long time. (I was too hardened by the continuous pain over the years to cry.) I stood there in his arms, beginning to relax, my head now resting on his shoulder, beginning to feel safe. Just like I did all those years ago in Galway when my mom came into the hotel room to hold me. I began to think maybe things would be ok, maybe I will be ok. It was the most perfect response from him, no words, no advice, just the hug; the showing of loving support, which helped me that day, to unmask a little more.

If I believe someone is suicidal then I will ask them straight out, 'Are you thinking about suicide?' I would not worry that I'm going to put the thought into their head. As with me, it was already there, a constant thought.

If you don't ask then you'll never know, and not be able to help. And if they open up to you, you can't promise you won't tell someone else, be it a parent or a manager or a doctor.

I made massive strides on that life-changing Monday morning. What stays with me most is the realisation that I do have people who care about me and who love me very much. They were there all the time, but I was so blinded by depression, I couldn't see it. That day I learned to feel the love, and I learned to accept physical contact, something I hadn't realised I'd shied away from or even missed for that matter. This love is not unique to me, you also have it in your life, you just need to allow yourself to see it!

Okay so, but I'm doing it for you guys!

After the hug we went to the kitchen and I finally had that cup of coffee. Paul informed me that he'd called Pieta House on the way home and they agreed to see me straight away, if I wanted to attend. I wasn't upset that he'd taken this action because I still had the choice to go or not. He had called them to have options open, so that action could be taken as soon as possible, if that's what I chose to do. Paul did the right thing. He created options for me. I could stay with Paul and Sinead and talk from there, or I could go with them to Pieta House and get further help. It was good to have support options available for myself but also for Paul and Sinead, as this was very much an unknown for them.

As I mentioned previously, there are no rules governing how family and friends will react. Paul called Pieta House without consulting me, which the majority of the time I would say is a no- no, because it should have been my decision, or at the very least, we should have discussed it. This unilateral decision could have driven me away and closed me off again. I'm not alone in this; many of us who suffer from depression or anxiety still believe we know what is best for us, which we don't. If we did, we would have taken positive action already, to help ourselves. Our mental health problems effectively control us, making us powerless, and suddenly control is being taken away once more, by other people.

Although, the seriousness of the situation should be taken into account. Even though I would have been against going to a place such as Pieta House. We have to realise sometimes family and friends take matters into their own hands out of love and respect. I now think Paul did the right thing. No, of course he did; it continued the knock-on effect of me taking action to manage my crippling mental health problems.

So, I was sitting at the kitchen table, cradling my coffee as if it was a comfort blanket, and looking out into their back garden. Paul asked, would I go to Pieta House to meet with them and see if they can work with me. My response was a resounding NO! I still felt great from my initial talk, and opening up to my family had been an exhausting step that morning. I didn't want others to know my situation, my weakness. I wasn't ready for that and I didn't want to go to a facility like *that*. It wasn't for me. I didn't need something like *that* (amazing how our mind works, right?). I didn't want people to look at me differently.

In fairness to my brother and Sinead, they didn't try to push me into anything. They just put some valid points across and made it sound like a good idea to just chat with a professional, and if I didn't like it, I could always leave. Yes, I did harbour fears of not being able to leave, being checked into some facility somewhere. I really didn't know what to expect, but eventually, albeit reluctantly, I agreed to go, with the assurance that I could leave at any time. You might be saying to yourself, YES, well done Neil, but hold that thought a second. I agreed to go, not for me, but for them. I agreed to go for my family. I was still not buying into it! What was the point?

Recognising is not accepting

With those words, 'Okay, so, but only for you,' I was really still not accepting my mental health problems. I wasn't accepting that I needed help. Non-acceptance can be a denial of your depression, of your anxiety. Your thinking might be that if you accept it, then it's a sign of weakness. Totally untrue! Accepting something so frightening and uncertain, and then taking action shows real courage and real strength! Believe me.

Yes, I knew there was something not right with me, but I never labelled myself as having mental health problems. That was something others had, like those movies with the psychiatric wards and patients wandering aimlessly about the corridors. That most certainly wasn't me. I just didn't fit in with this life. Therefore, I wasn't going to Pieta House for me, as I knew, in my great wisdom, that it would not work. I was doing it for others. I was doing it out of courtesy for Paul and Sinead; sure, hadn't they helped me that morning? I mean WTF, Neil! So, no, I wasn't accepting my problems as mental health. I wasn't accepting the fact that anyone outside of myself could help me.

I had recognised my problems from an early age (15-years-old), that I was 'different' from other people. I *realised* that something wasn't quite right. However, I did not *accept* that it was my mental health. Accepting that was difficult. I didn't know how to accept it. I didn't want to show weakness, nobody does. I didn't want to instigate a process of going to this doctor or that, or whatever the procedure was for this kinda thing. It would change everything if I were to accept it. Things would never go back to the way they were (Eh, that'd be a good thing, right?). Easier to help myself the only way I know how, and don my mask each and every time it was necessary. This act of masking distanced me from opportunities to seek help.

Recognising when something is not right with you is a great skill to have, but an even better one is taking action. Act, don't brush it under the carpet and hope it goes away. That's kinda like when you were a kid in school and the teacher was calling on students to answer questions. So, you close your eyes in the daft hope that the teacher won't see you, and won't pick you to answer the question. Not gonna happen, right? More often than not, the teacher picks you. So, the more often you do this with your problems, the more likely they come back and present stronger than before.

The key to stepping onto a new path

Accepting your situation and accepting yourself with all your baggage is the key. Even after opening up about my mental health issues, I didn't truly accept my situation. I didn't accept me. Why the hell would I, right? Accept all that shit and have to deal with it; eh, no thanks, I'll stay the way I am.

When I analyse that, staying within a state of denial kinda meant I thought I would be happier living with my darkness, my constant struggle, and thoughts of wanting to die. And this was better than looking in a mirror and accepting my reality?

I had to change this way of thinking. Turn my attention to acceptance rather than the so-called comfort zone of denial. What if I accepted the pain I was going through? Would it have allowed me to deal with my problems more effectively? I very much feel it would. Now, today, I can say it has. Accepting it opened me up to more opportunities to help myself, allowed me to not have to deal with it alone. I accepted that my mental health problems were very much part of me, I stopped this charade of denying which blocked me from being able to find new ways to deal with the pain and struggle.

As we know, for me, talking was a crucial action. Combine that with acceptance, and I'm more open and willing to keep on talking and sharing and opening up. This acceptance allows more exploration into my mental health problems, which in turn feeds into a more well-rounded plan, which you can put in place to deal with the problems, and find the real you again. How cool is that?

Think about it this way. You love your family, right? You love your friends? You love them unconditionally, the way they are, their talents, their presence, their caring and much more. You also love them despite their vulnerabilities, or, if you like, what you perceive as their inadequacies, right? Whatever they might be; they get angry quickly, they are messy, they are shy in public; whatever it is, you still love them to pieces, because you accept them in their entirety. Knowing the 'full' someone and still loving them is acceptance. You have no problem with this, it seems natural for you, you don't question it. So why can we not do the same for ourselves and especially when suffering from mental health problems? Why do we block it and deny it?

You might be thinking, I do accept my problems and myself now as I am. That might be true to a certain extent, but let me ask you this. Do you still mask it in certain situations? Are there times when you don't talk about it, and endure it alone rather than open up? Do people outside your family know about it? Does work know about it? Does the person you're dating know about it?

I know I still mask it at times. Those times when I still don't talk, those times when I meet new people, those times when the easier option for me is to stay silent. But I'm getting better at this acceptance thing as each day passes. The difference between me, now, and Neil of the past, is that I know I have the tools in place to call on when I'm low or anxious. These tools I use every day, not only to manage myself when I'm low or anxious, but to maintain my state of good mental health.

When you fully accept yourself and your problems, you've taken the most important step towards moving onto a new path and being able to manage your problems effectively. It's the most important because it will enable you to strive for sustainable 'good' mental health. You will come to accept your depression and anxiety and the things which might trigger them. You accept there might be tough times ahead but you're now in a better position to deal with it. Acceptance will help you to become more resilient. When you accept it, and yourself, you'll be more open to learning about yourself, and gain a better understanding of what you're going through. It will allow you to free your mind from the hold it has over you, which will enable you to focus your attention elsewhere.

If you keep denying it, which essentially is fighting it, everything feels like a battle; hard to get out of bed, hard to stay alert, hard to work and hard to relax.

The great thing here is you have a choice: Continue as you are or choose to accept yourself in your entirety. This does not mean you're giving in to your depression or anxiety, and resigning yourself to the fact that this is just the way it is. It means you're now listening to yourself, taking on board how things are affecting you.

Now you're ready to help yourself.

Chapter 14
A shift in thinking

A shift in thinking! What did you say? I had to shift and change my default thinking pattern, one which has been in-built for the best part of three decades. This was very much going to be an uphill battle. Changing my negative thoughts to ones of more positive a nature.

This does not mean being positive all the time. It means changing how you think about situations you might find yourself in. I'm not alone in this; most of us unleash the negativity first. What I, and maybe you also, do, is tend to hang on to the negative reaction instead of trying to kick it to the curb and change our reaction to a more positive one. So, I had to realise that even when I unleashed a negative reaction it was still possible for me to change it.

Positive thoughts are more difficult to muster. They do take work, especially at the beginning of this new process, but there is always a positive thought you can muster in any situation. The key, as with everything new we learn, is being consistent. You have to become very aware and recognise when the negative thought has arrived and then consciously change to replace it with a positive one.

Negative thoughts can consume me when something as non-threatening as an email arrives to my inbox. I automatically think it's something bad. If it's for work, I think it's an email cancelling my contract, or that the company wants to have a meeting about my work, as they are not happy with me. Which leads me to not opening the email. I don't want to face this truth that I've told myself, but instead I will visit and revisit my inbox many more times before I strike up the courage to open it. There is no escape from this email and the bowl of negative thoughts it has served up.

More often than not the email is something as simple as wanting to confirm my bank details or thanking me for the work I've done so far. I've wasted a heap of time fretting about its content because my mind unleashes the negative thought pattern, which spirals out of control as I decline to open the email. I was worried and stressed over nothing. Imagine, if I could change this thought pattern, I would have opened the email and saved myself the trouble and emotional roller-coaster I forced myself through. Now I face an uphill battle to kickstart my day and turn this anxiety on its head.

Neil's Notes

There are many simple tools I've utilised in order to shift my negative thoughts. If you're up for it, try this:

Each time your brain turns to a negative thought after some conflict or dissonance in work or a relationship, try to recognise that you're having a negative thought, and switch it to a positive thought and reaction instead. This can be done by trying to find the positive in the situation.

1. Is the thought the truth?
2. How do I know it is?
3. Where's the evidence?
4. What are the pro's for me thinking like this?
5. What are the con's for me thinking like this?

    6.   What's the worst that can happen?

    7.   What's the best that could happen?

What you're trying to do is get yourself acquainted with what's going on in your head? Catch it, and flip it.

— ◆ —

I'm still powerless

I felt powerless when depression or anxiety took hold. I was at their mercy and there wasn't a thing I could do. They (depression or anxiety, known as D&A) would strike when they saw fit and I had to adjust to their demands. I have, in the past, cancelled clients, meetings, courses and even activities I arranged and enjoyed, like meeting friends because D&A had struck me down. Once I felt them claiming me, I would know that my day was a non-runner and whatever I had planned was out of the window.

In the morning, if I woke up to find body and mind taken over by D&A, I would sit up in bed, take the phone out and text a lie to my clients. Well, a fabrication of the truth, that I was down with the flu and felt really unwell or some bullshit like that. The reply from the client or friends would be one of understanding and concern, making me feel even worse. My day was cancelled.

I might lie in bed on day one, day two, day three. No contact, thoughts swirling, body aching with no end in sight. But I always managed to wait it out, taking shelter under the covers. Therein lay the problem. I was doing something (waiting it out and taking shelter) which was of no benefit to me whatsoever. During a storm you can stay inside taking shelter from the elements, be safe and comfortable. When the mental health storm hits, there is no such shelter or comfort. Covering my head with a duvet, trying to hide does not stop the storm inside my head or the physical shake in the body. It does not help in changing the inevitability of future storms again down the line. Does this sound familiar to you? Are you constantly trying to seek new ways to just survive this continuous never-ending cycle of the storm? To just get through it?

I found myself, even after seeking support, still defaulting, taking shelter and waiting out the storm. How futile was that? It was of no benefit, either before the episode hit, or during the inner chaos. I was like a cowboy holding onto a bucking horse for dear life, knowing if I fell off worse pain awaits me.

At this stage I had also started my weekly counselling session with Pieta House. These sessions, although beneficial, also fed into my reluctance to address a storm. I would endure the struggle and leave it until the counselling relieved me of the turmoil. I'd *only* have to wait and survive a couple of days. Such an irrational process on my part. Not even trying to take matters into my own hands. The truth of the matter is, to endure this storm, if even for a minute is too long and could have more damaging consequences in the long run.

Actually, get this right! Even when people knew about me and my situation, even when I knew I had support around me, I didn't open up to them anymore. The reason for this failure of mine, opening up to people again, was because I now had a professional counsellor helping, and, according to the bible of Neil's mind, I should not be selfish and drag my family and friends into my little storms anymore.

Oh Neil, Oh Neil, Oh Neil, what will we do with you, eh?

Life behind that mask wasn't easy to shed. Little did I know that very soon I would come to realise I had the power within me to turn my life around. All I had to do was access it.

Counselling won't work for me

I followed the lady down the hall to a large room with big windows looking out onto a driveway. I waited for my assessment. Thinking to myself, 'Well, I have nothing to share, nothing to say, this will be a complete waste of everyone's time.' My internal monologue was still the same, *I'm not stupid, people. Don't you know I've tried everything humanly possible to help myself?*' The assessment took place and, to be honest, I can't remember any of it. All I recall is that a counsellor would be appointed to me. So, my time at Pieta House had begun. I do remember thinking, 'What a waste of time this will be!'

The following week, I met my counsellor. I noticed, even before that first session, that I was in better form. The power of counselling, eh? I was already on my way to happiness before the first session had begun! I think it was the placebo effect of having wheels in motion to address my problems, coupled with the fact that I now had options of support. I didn't have to deal with my problems on my own anymore. But it was a short-term feeling.

I arrived at Pieta House for my first appointment with the counsellor, preferring to go alone. Going alone to the session was a massive step in itself. I could easily have backed out. I didn't have to go alone, as Paul offered to go with me, but I opted against it, mainly, I think, so as not to encroach on any more of his time. Looking back, it worked out okay, but if I were to retake this first session, I would have had someone accompany me.

I wasn't sure what to expect, and I knew this unknown could trigger my anxiety. This is something I should have tried to avoid at all costs. I should have put in place supports to help me get through the day. I didn't know how I would react to the session, whether I would find it too taxing mentally, and be an emotional wreck after, then have to drive home alone with my thoughts. Having someone with you can ease the anxiety and take away those extra unnecessary burdens.

I stood in the archway of the door, reminiscent of Will Smith standing at the door of his uncle's house during the opening credits of the TV show, 'The Fresh Prince of Bel Air', neither of us comprehending the potential for a new way to live, which lay behind our respective doors. Sadly, that's where the comparison with Will ends, he was filled with excitement and wonder, me with dread and hopelessness.

I ring the intercom at the door for access, enter, and sign-in at reception, with some unforgettable chit-chat as my eyes search for a seat. I spot one located away from prying eyes or potential conversation starters. I seat myself safely amongst others who are all, I presume, on a similar journey to mine albeit at various stages. While seated in the waiting room, thoughts flicker through my mind, ranging from devising a quick plan of escape and make it to the safety of my car and leave these people behind me, to thoughts of not liking my counsellor and feeling I've taken up a place for someone more worthy than I and who would find more benefit. These constant thoughts consuming me, I hide my gaze behind a Newsweek magazine.

'Neil.'

A short silence. 'Neil Kelders?'

I raise my gaze to find a woman waiting patiently. I stand and follow her down the hallway past some offices and into the room with the large window looking onto the driveway.

The lady closed the door behind me and offered me a seat. She sat and introduced herself as my assigned counsellor. Awkwardness ensued, followed by bouts of intermittent chat and silence. I felt uneasy throughout the session. I didn't warm to the counsellor. On quick reflection afterwards, I felt that it was a complete waste of time. And so I was justified in my belief before the session that it would be a waste of time. Whoop-de-doo Neil. What do you want: A bloody medal or something?

Week two: I arrive, ring the intercom, sign in, take a seat, follow a new lady to the room. A different counsellor. Not requested by me, but assigned by Pieta House. I'm glad they did because even though I wasn't happy with counsellor number one, I would have remained silent and not requested another. Therefore, continuing with a process that was only going to amount to a negative experience for me. If this happened then counselling would have been black-marked by me for good. Do you know what that would mean in reality? It means I would have just closed the door on a potential lifesaving opportunity, thus narrowing my chances of successfully dealing with my problems.

We sat, we talked, we stayed silent. We talked again; we said our goodbyes. This time as I drove away, I reflected on the session. Much happier! Not that we explored much, but I felt a better connection and more comfortable with this counsellor.

Weekly sessions continued, with periods of talking broken up with moments of silence. I was becoming more comfortable and willing to participate in the sessions, so those silences were becoming less as time went by. We explored my problems, highlighted areas I could work on and I continuously learned about myself and life in general. I like to think that we learned from each other. You see, I like to analyse theories or reasons or opinions or anything really. I would discuss my thoughts of things like the statement, 'It's okay not to be okay.' What really appealed to me was that my counsellor was open to such discussions. What was even more appealing to me was the fact that if she did not know something or how to answer something then she would say so. She was open and honest (as I was trying to be), and would go away for the week and come back to the next session informed on the points I had made, also having formed an opinion of her own. She made me feel valid and seemed genuinely interested in my thoughts, ideas and story. You might think this is nothing to write home about. Isn't that a counsellor's job you might ask? Yes, it is indeed. A counsellor's job is to do all of that, but you get some who are better at it than others. It's all well and good having knowledge and education, but that needs to be complemented with people skills and the art of listening and understanding the person sitting in front of you.

You won't connect with all counsellors or psychiatrists you have dealings with. Read that line again, it's important. They are people, like you and me; some we like and connect with and some we don't. I knew this was the counsellor for me. From my experience with this second counsellor, I knew counselling could now play an important role for me and my development.

How have your counselling experiences been? Have you ever had any? If you have, take a moment to write down what was positive and negative about the experience. What stands out for you? Next time you go to a counsellor, instead of going through the motions and finding the process a waste of time, which is something I've heard from friends and clients alike, put ideas forward to the counsellor sitting in front of you, say what you want from the sessions and what you don't want. Remember counselling sessions are your sessions, they're about you. You can have an input on how to shape them.

People regularly tell me they wouldn't go to counselling; it wouldn't or hasn't worked for them, 'Yeah, you know it's not for me because all they do is have you talk and talk with no real advice, no real structure.' People say that their previous experiences with counsellors were poor, that it felt like the counsellor was going through the motions and just wanted the money with no real interest in the client. Some stories people have relayed to me, about some counselling experiences have been, I would say, horrific.

During one session, a counsellor said to her client, '*I don't know what to say to you, I can't help you with that,*' and a second one, where the counsellor said to the client, 'You're *wrecking my head.*' I know it's hard to believe that this happened, but unfortunately it did. Do you realise how damaging that can be to that person sitting in front of the counsellor, never mind how unprofessional it is.

I have learned, as someone people come to for support, that there is a decorum when making yourself available. I have to be careful when interacting one to one, when doing face-to-face talks or webinars, when posting on social media. I make sure I listen without judgement, that I guide the people to ideas that might help them, that I provide sound knowledge backed with my personal experience.

Even while writing this book, I have to be conscious of you, the reader, to remember that we are all at different stages in our journey, and I'm not in your shoes. I can't tell you that you'll overcome your mental health problems. What I can tell you and show you is that you can live with them and manage them effectively, with limited disruption to your daily journey. I have to remember that my words and actions can have a lasting impression, as do counsellors. Words matter and more, so when dealing with people who are more than likely going to be quite vulnerable, my role is to steer you away from the negative, the self-doubt, the lack of hope, and unleash the more positive and hopeful mindset.

Yes, as in every other profession, there are counsellors who are not as good, not as clued in, not a people person; some you might even describe as being a joke. They are people, right? Male or female, the counsellor or psychiatrist is a person just like you and me, and some people are just bad at their job. Even if they are good, they might just not be the right fit for you. Think of, say, a personal trainer. If you don't click or connect with your personal trainer, what do you do? You find a new one. You don't give up exercise altogether, do you? It's exactly the same with a counsellor: Find the right one for you, and don't settle for one you feel isn't working for you. Be honest with your assessment. Make sure you're assessing their performance from a position of stability and not when consumed by a low, or anxiety. Make sure you have realistic expectations; many of us attend counselling expecting our lives to be changed overnight. This won't happen. It's a process that will awaken something new in you and help redirect your mindset and create some hope. Give the process some time as there is always bound to be some settling-in period. After you've given this counsellor a fair shot, and still feel they are not for you, then by all means find another. Sometimes counsellors come recommended, but that doesn't mean they will be 'great' for you. But don't stop the counselling process. Don't have a period of a total cessation of counselling, search for a new one while still attending the current sessions.

Do not give up on this process. Excuse me! Did you hear me? Please don't give up on it. Find the counsellor for you!

She really understood me

I was initially assigned, I think, fifteen counselling sessions.

As I was 'a risk' I started with two sessions per week. I continued attending, even though at times, I doubted that this process would work and so wasn't fully committed. Having this lack of hope and confidence that anything I ever did could change my current situation being part and parcel of my mental health problems.

There were many days, as I drove to my session, when that feeling of dread would come over me and stay with me right up until the moment I sat in the counsellor's chair, every moment wanting to text and cancel my session. Thankfully I resisted all urges. Showing up for the session, walking in the door of the counsellor's office, was a win for me. It's just so easy to say no. It's so easy to cancel and, as you know, it's so easy to sabotage ourselves, which I did time and again throughout my life. So, this was definitely a win, just that little step of walking in the door each week.

Now, to build on that was key.

During the sessions we would talk and I often felt I had contributed nothing. I was so closed, and of course the fact that I'm astute didn't help, as I would not fall for any tricks she employed when trying to open me up. I knew what I didn't want to happen in the session. I didn't want her to look at me as 'poor Neil,' and I wanted to avoid having these sessions all about my childhood and father leaving us, blah blah blah. I was sick of going over that in my head, and I believed I had come to terms with that years ago. I knew that if she was to really help me, I needed a bloody challenge and not this gentle chat bull.

When I look back on it, there are a few things that really stood out for me with this counsellor. The first was that, around session two or three, she told me that she was going to have to challenge me – bingo! – safely challenge me of course. I hadn't mentioned to her that this is what I wanted, but after two sessions of observing and listening, I felt like she understood me. It blew my mind. This felt like the first time someone had 'got me' in a very long time. The connection and trust was being built.

The second thing that really stood out was how honest she was. As I said, I like to analyse things and dig deep and give my ideas around a topic or a point. Take the example of the statement I gave earlier, 'It's okay not to be okay.' Another example would be my take on talking. Where we are told it's good to talk, but the fact of the matter it's not that easy. She would take it on board and if it made her question her ideas or if she didn't have an answer, she would say so and would come back to the next session having thought about our conversation, and share her understanding of what I was saying. My sessions were extended for another ten or so, so yeah, I suppose twenty-one years of suppression does need a lot of exploration and challenging.

The third thing that stands out was something she said towards the end of our sessions. 'Neil, I think we have to look at our sessions, I feel I can't take you for counselling anymore, that you're not engaged in the sessions, and are giving the answers you think I want to hear.' Shit, she got me. She was totally right. I had, for at least the last two sessions, started to disengage. I was still participating and remained active in the sessions, but only so as to mask my change in feeling about our sessions.

She was very much tuned-in, and *noticed* me.

I was amazed to be honest. This highlighted even further that she really did understand me, she was interested in me and wasn't afraid to put up her hand and say, 'I can't take you any further.' What really surprised me was that she put her ego aside and admitted that it was time for me to be passed to someone else. She made the sessions about me, not about her. This also proves that my journey is a continuous one, as are all of our journeys in this life. We should never stop learning. It made me a little sad thinking about not coming back to this counsellor, because I would be leaving behind someone who 'got me'.

I would have to move out of the comfort zone I had established over the last number of weeks and progress to the next step on my journey. But this is what life is about. To experience it to the max, you have to keep moving forward and out of those comfort zones we constantly find ourselves in.

My sessions with this counsellor played a major role in where I am today. Her professionalism, her genuine care, honesty and her understanding of me, brought me back into this world that I felt was no longer for me. I now feel that there are people in this life who will understand me, who will care about me, even perfect strangers. People who will take time to help me, who will be honest with me and not judge me. These sessions with my counsellor had helped me create a greater self-acceptance and an inner strength to fight for my life.

As I contemplated working with a new counsellor, one recommended by the last one, something dawned on me, an epiphany if you like, which was about to change my life and way of thinking even further: I would have to start taking responsibility. Not easy to hear, I know, but I had to win from within! I made the bold decision to not opt for another counsellor and try to find ways to help myself.

Chapter 15
Whose responsibility?

Yes, you've read that correctly. I know it's the last thing you want to hear; it was the last thing I wanted to hear. 'You are telling me that you want me to take responsibility and I feel like this? I'm at the bottom of the blackest, darkest hole you can imagine, shit's being poured on me, and YOU want me to take responsibility, you asshole.' Yup! I think it's so important to take responsibility. But only when the time is right. If you're sitting there now, having accepted your situation, and have already sought help (by the way, by you reading this book, that's a version of seeking help), then you've started taking some responsibility. But there is more you can do for yourself, there always is. There is this untapped power within you. Yes, and I know responsibility can seem to be an unforgiving term, but in essence, that's what it is. You taking responsibility is accessing the power within you. It's time to access your power which means it's time to activate your ability to manage your mental health problems.

I have a little analogy for you! Ah, come on, humour me! Okay, so let's say you're studying for an exam. You have acquired the best supports possible to help you get the best result possible. This may be: Having the best teacher or lecturer, taking the best notes from class, having the best peer study group, employing the best tutor, having an understanding family who create an amazing study environment for you, creating the best study plan, as well as all the other top class supports that are available to you. All are amazing and will surely help you with the exam, right? But can you think of anything which might reduce the effectiveness of these supports. Now let's say you skip class on regular occasions and have no understanding of the course content, as you don't read the notes given in each class. Now, I ask you how effective the support will be? Yes, they can help but now their energies will have to go into bringing you up to speed on course content. Now as the exam fast approaches they might need to focus on getting you the pass in the exam rather the best result possible.

But if you took responsibility and attended class and made sure you took good notes and read and studied them, then those supports would have been able to put more energy into getting you a much better result in the exam. By you taking responsibility, those supports you have in place for the exam could really propel you forward. So, a combination of the outside supports and you taking this responsibility will guarantee a better result.

Link that logic to your mental health problems. This is what I realised I had to do: When it was time to move counsellors, I made the decision to respectfully decline and start the process of finding ways for me to work on myself. (A very important point of note here. I only did this when I felt ready. I would recommend continuing with a counsellor while you explore taking this responsibility, and even when you're stronger and more confident, it's always good to have a counsellor as a resource). I was in a stronger position now than ever before. But I felt there were holes in the current process. For example, during my time at Pieta House, when I would experience a very low period or my anxiety would cripple me, I would think that it would be okay once I saw my counsellor. But sometimes the appointment could be five days away, especially towards the end, as we only saw each other once a week! So, I would endure the lows and anxiety until my session with the counsellor. How sustainable was that going to be?

How long could I keep doing that for? Wouldn't that mean that each individual counselling session would only be putting out fires rather than being progressive and explorative?

Don't get me wrong, the support was great. The counselling, the talking, the assistance around me, but I had nothing really in place to help me in that exact moment of my darkness. That is when the penny dropped. If I was to be able to move out of this cycle and manage it effectively, while living the life I wanted, then I would have to take some responsibility to manage my problems. It's a more positive way to think about it. Taking responsibility can be daunting, but accessing your power tells you that *you* have the strength to do this, yourself.

Accessing my power has been essential for me in attaining a sustainable good mental health. The beauty about empowering myself is that I now have the means at my disposal to help myself when I feel low. I now have the means to help me maintain that good mental health for more prolonged periods of time. This power is not only to help ease the pain of my struggles but also there to maintain the good times, which makes it more difficult for my depression and anxiety to paralyse me.

Accessing your power is a continuous process

My next question was, how the hell am I going to access my own power? Where do I even start? It eventually dawned on me that I had already begun this process. It began that day in April when I talked. It hadn't clicked with me back then. There was no way I would have thought that I was 'accessing my power' on that day.

To access it I had to become vulnerable, to myself and to others, and this vulnerability allowed me to open up. I had to be okay with lowering the mask. Yes, it had been lowered a few times already but I needed to continue to do it and not second-guess myself. I had to accept that my mental health problems are a part of me. They don't define me but are very much a part of me, as yours are to you.

No black dog here

Terms you'll often hear communicated when people offer descriptions of depression are: It hangs like a black cloud over you, or it's as if a black dog is constantly following you. Accepting that my depression, anxiety and suicidal ideation are part of my current make-up meant that I didn't have to subscribe to these terms. If I were to use these expressions in relation to my mental health, then I would be externalising it. By that I mean, I would then believe that my mental health problems are not part of me but something external. If I were to believe this then I would not think the tools or action steps I've developed to manage my problems would be as useful or successful. Externalising my problems would mean I see them as separate to me, that I have no connection to them.

I can understand why people think this way. I mean, who wants to acknowledge something so terrible as being a part of them? If I externalised them, it would therefore mean I wasn't accepting that I had some mental health problems, well, not to the fullest extent anyway. But if I see these issues as part of me, I internalise them, and by doing this I can actually have some control over the extent to which the problems affect me. If I internalise my issues, believe they are part of me, I'm able to recognise and become familiar with features of my depression and anxiety; that feeling when episodes are incoming, identify what triggers them, and connect to what I need to do to keep my head above water on those bad days. It is, as they say, better the devil you know than the devil you don't.

If you keep identifying your issues as external to you (black dog, black cloud etc), then you don't really have any mastery over yourself. You will more than likely find yourself being reactive rather than pro-active when managing your problems; trying to outrun your problems and beat them away. This can work to a degree, but how long can you keep up with that intensity? What happens on the day when you can't outrun your externalised problems? What will you do then? I know what happened to me. They floored me. They gave me the beating. I was powerless. All I could ever do was try as best as I could to weather the storm, knowing it wouldn't be the last.

I'm making nice progress here. So far, I've started to take responsibility, I've come to see my mental health problems as part of me, internal rather than external. Now is a good time to go exploring ways and means to manage this part of me. What things will I introduce into my life that will be of benefit to me when I'm going through a dark episode? And what can I introduce to help me maintain and prolong those periods of stability?

Neil da explora

Let's get stuck in. Early on I realised I had no real structure, or if I had put one in place, I did not follow it for too long. All planning and no follow through, that's me!

I need a structure; we all do. But I need one which I will stick to, if it's too structured and intense then it will fall apart, or more than likely, I will. It will overwhelm me, for sure. I identified that my mornings are all over the place and the morning is the time that feeds my whole day. So, first stop is a morning routine.

What can I do to set myself up for my day? Well, I do know that the minute I open my eyes it's very easy for my mind to go to the negative. So, I need to find ways to counteract this. A morning routine in itself will have my mind more focused as I now have some tasks or as I prefer to label them; little wins.

My routine is personal to me. When the alarm sounds in the morning, I jump out of bed instead of pressing the snooze button. I then drink water from the bottle I've placed beside my bed the night before. I make my bed. All very simple steps but for me I now have three wins already bagged at the start of my day. Then I meditate, as it allows me to proceed with my day with a calmer, clearer head. I review my daily plan. Next up is exercise, which for me is best in the morning times. I get lazy in the evenings.

All of these make up my morning wins. Wins are achievements that make me feel good about myself. They ensure a positive mindset as I move on with my day. Yes, of course I can still have a bad day, but these morning wins, combined with my evening routine, filled with more wins, means I'm giving myself a fighting chance and a better platform from which to face any problems.

I view these morning and evening routines as part of my workday or as an important component of a productive Neil day. That is why I call activities like meditation and exercise non-negotiables. I treat them like an important meeting which I can't reschedule. I exercise and meditate in the early mornings because I know me, and I'm less likely to exercise later in the day, no matter how much I promise myself.

Even with such great routines in place, I have the odd day where I can feel my darkness returning. This was so frustrating at first, because I had worked hard on developing these routines. So, why the hell am I dipping? Ready to give up and feel nothing was going to work for me. When I eventually allowed myself to be less hard on myself, I realised that all of us have slow starts to some days, or our form can dip at any time. This is life, and not just me. So, yes at times I might still become a little anxious or low. Knowing this, I had to turn my focus to acquiring steps to manage these situations.

No rules apply!

Never stop learning about yourself. That is my advice, plain and simple. You need to really take your time and be patient when looking for tools that will help you on this journey. Be creative. Be inventive. Look at everything as a possible tool. There are no rules or steps to follow. This is for you, made by you.

My favourite is the 'burning of my worries'. Simply put, it's where I write down, without thinking what is swirling around in my head. A brain dump, if you like. I don't stop writing to think or review what I've written. I just get all those very random, nonsensical thoughts out of my head and onto paper.

My mind becomes less heavy and is tricked into thinking that maybe I've addressed all those outstanding thoughts. I don't read the paper but I fold it over, tear it up and throw it away or, more dramatically, burn it. I then move on with my day.

The point is I can call on this tool to help me at any time, even when I'm being consistent with my daily routine and things still go pear-shaped. It's important to remember that even though you follow all the right steps to help yourself, you will still at times feel like crap. This knowledge, combined with the tools or power I've built up, ensure that I'm ready and able to take the responsibility needed to help myself, and don't default to a defeated state. I hope that makes sense to you?

Look within

This internalisation of my mental health problems, as previously stated, has allowed me to become familiar with my depression and anxiety. It allows me to know how they affect both my body and mind so that I can adapt to the influence they have, and still be functional and productive.

Remember the descriptions I gave earlier in the book as to what depression and anxiety felt like, physically? Well, I was able to express it with such vivid imagery because having internalised my problems, I was able to connect and feel its impact on my body. I can now recognise an impending attack. Feeling it not only in mind, but also in body; thereby allowing me to take immediate action, before it develops into a full-blown attack. This was me being proactive rather than remaining reactive.

This is the step you want to take; this is where you can still see the beauty in life past all the darkness. Once I had taken the action steps of talking, accepting, and internalising my depression and anxiety, I then had to explore and scan through my arsenal of tools as to which could help me when my depression or anxiety hit. If you're suffering from the dreaded depression and anxiety, or even stress, try one or two of them for yourself and see how they work for you.

Time to dig!

To make sure I was making the most of my newfound power, I then had to try to focus on reflection. I needed access to objective feedback (this is done when stability is resumed) after a bout of depression or anxiety, to discover what I believed triggered this episode, explore how I reacted to the situation, and recall what tools had worked to counter it, and which didn't work so well this time around.

I would objectively look at various areas of my life and work, the people and relationships, and re-evaluate the point or purpose I had found for my life.

This reflection allowed me to find the best tools for me to integrate into daily life, which I had to maybe tweak or adapt to meet my specific need. Which tools worked best to maintain stability, and which worked better when in the midst of an episode. It highlighted if I needed to update my database of tools.

Reflection is a powerful tool, as it frequently highlights when I have to make important decisions in order to progress on my new path. It will remind me time and again that episodes arise because I have not acted to make the necessary changes, therefore those triggers distort my path.

Reflecting on episodes and problematic situations has led me to put myself first instead of always choosing to not upset others, which I would do even if it adversely affected me.

Chapter 16
Changes - a show of strength!

I chose me. The moment I decided to choose myself above anything else was pivotal. I needed to look after myself, because I knew if I didn't, I would rebound back to the Neil before that Monday morning on 14th April 2014.

The time had arrived for me to make some tough decisions; some more difficult than others, but all necessary. I looked at those people who made me feel like shit, and dumped their arses! I began to assess my relationships with the people around me. I knew those who drained me, especially those people who dumped constant negativity my way. Some people have negativity seeping from pores. You know the ones; if the sun is splitting the stones, they don't acknowledge the lovely day but comment that it will rain soon. They can't enjoy the moment.

People. I chose carefully. In 2008 I worked for a company in Co. Kerry. At the time I was studying law in the next county over, Co. Cork. I would arrive into work quite early each morning in order to be allowed to leave early for my long drive ahead for college in the evenings.

I enjoyed the couple hours in the office to myself. No distractions and very productive. A colleague would then arrive into the office, usually around 8.15am. I would down-tools for a well-deserved break and we would go to the cafe next door. I did enjoy this woman's company, initially. After some time, that opinion slowly faded. Every word out of her mouth was negative. If she wasn't complaining about some colleague, she was complaining about the weather or giving out about some impending changes in work.

It began to eat away at me, and I no longer enjoyed the morning coffee but, guess what? I continued to go. Why? Just out of sheer politeness and not wanting to offend her. Damn fool that I was, I should have nipped it in the bud. Listening to this negativity each morning definitely impacted on me for the day, and as you know, I wasn't in the best shape myself at this time. Her negativity compounded mine and sunk me a little deeper into my darkness. I should have politely declined her offers. This I now have the strength to do. If something doesn't sit right with me, then I will decline offers of connection and move on with my day, week and life. Sorry but I come first now! This colleague wasn't a bad person and someone else might not even have noticed her negativity, but I had, and I needed to do what was right for me.

Relationships. There are others out there who are just toxic, who didn't treat me with the respect I accorded them; relationships that gave nothing back to me. The relationship was on their terms, connecting and meeting when suited them. Those relationships drained me, especially when I was younger, as I would bend over backwards not to offend, and hope to be included. Those relationships involved both friendships and dating, and essentially just ended up with me feeling shit about myself.

Work: I quit work. Yes, I had bills to pay, a mortgage and all the rest but my work was contributing to my poor mental health. I chose me. Not many people will take a close look at how their job is stressing them; how it consumes their days; how it affects their weekend, not being able to let deadlines or workloads go, constantly thinking of the coming week.

Where I live. I moved. I had a house in a village called Milltown, which was a 15-minute drive from my home town of Killarney. I bought the house in 2004 with my then girlfriend. We broke up in 2008, and I had no ties to or connection to the area. I longed to leave the house and venture further afield. But fear had blocked me for years. I relocated. It felt right and like a good decision to move to Dublin city. Even if I wasn't quite sure what I was getting myself into. When a business opportunity in the big city didn't work out as planned, I surprised myself and stayed put, not falling backwards and heading back down South to Kerry and the comfort of home.

Passions. I made time. I decided I wanted to embrace my running life once again. This was at a time when I was trying hard to beat my depressive episodes. I looked at the changes or actions which I could take to realise this new goal. I had to accept that I was starting out again and needed to keep the focus on myself, not what others around me were doing or posting in social media about their running exploits.

So, I made changes that worked for me and, believe me, you'll think these minute steps ridiculous, but this was about me and how I could achieve my goal. You might discover a different path.

Day one I changed into my running gear and just walked around the house, stopping on occasion to stretch. I'm serious. I knew I wasn't ready to hit the streets as my mind would work against me from the off, and put me off this reintroduction of running. The second day I put on my gear again. This time I put on my runners and went out-side to walk around my estate. Day three and I did as I had done the previous day but this time I went for a run. This gives you an idea of the minute changes I had to make in order to change my mindset, to do what was best for me, no matter how foolish or idiotic it might have looked to an outsider.

Not all the changes I introduced into my life were so extreme. Most were simple to help me day to day. I changed the time I woke up in the mornings. I changed my morning routine. I introduced meditation to my day. I stopped drinking coffee at night time. All simple but effective.

My favourite quote, espoused by many but inspired originally by the great Albert Einstein, is, '*If you do nothing, then nothing changes*', and I add to the words, 'Do something'. I repeat this constantly. I use it to sign off from videos, webinars, workshops, online courses, even this book. It hit home that I needed to just start making the smallest of changes if I was to have any hope of actually living my life.

Neil's Notes

Change, no matter how big or small, is hard. It can be hard for anyone, not to mind those of us struggling with some mental health problems. In order to find the resolve to make these life-changing decisions, I had to ask myself some key questions. These are questions you can ask yourself right now. Think about the last time you felt low, stressed or anxious. Explore the situation by asking the following:

- When I felt at my worst, was there a pattern in how I reacted to or dealt with it?
- Did something trigger it? Is this trigger common to most or all previous situations?
- What could I do to stabilise myself? Do I need introduce something new, remove something or replace something in my day, week, life?
- How could I still be somewhat productive and not end up in bed in darkness?
- How can I make this change I've identified without causing myself more conflict or overwhelm?

Stop reading, please. Explore one change you can make right now! It's time to act!

—◆—

Change is important!

If you asked me, 'Neil what changes could I make to help myself?' I would tell you that only you can truly answer that. Yes, I can guide you, give you ideas, open you up to change, but only you can find what really works for you. However, if you pushed me into answering, I would tell you to find ways to stay in the here and now. Be present in the moment and when you feel your mind wandering, recognise it and bring it back here. To this day I continue to find new ways to ground myself in the moment, because yes, my mind can still wander. It happens to us all.

Be kind to yourself. This was actually something my counsellor highlighted. I was so hard on myself, over the smallest of things. This reaction would disrupt my whole day. I bet you can be hard on yourself?

I had to realise that some days were going to be more challenging than others and, you know what? That's okay. It's also okay to rethink and adapt my plans and hopes for those days I wasn't feeling well. I had to accept that the goal had shifted, and it was more important for me to look after myself rather than get lost while trying to achieve my plan.

Being kinder to myself also meant that if anxiety was gripping me, I would stop what I was doing and, without feeling guilty, get up and move, get some air and change my focus. These changes meant I was now aware that it was acceptable for me to feel this way (low or anxious) and that it was important to look after number one.

Support. Always be open to it. I'm more open to drawing on new supports, be it in the form of family members, friends, online groups and courses, as well as chatting with those whose stories were similar to mine.

I was open to exploring new supports and, more importantly, to the fact that not everything I adopted would suit me or be of real benefit. I knew a tool or support could be adapted and shaped to meet my specific needs. That could be doing just a five-minute exercise session instead of the 30 minutes or an hour. Doing five minutes of meditation instead of 20 minutes or attending my counsellor once every two weeks instead of once or twice a week. The goal wasn't for me to simply acquire a collection of supports and tools, but to sculpt them into tools which benefited me personally, ones I knew I would utilise. Adding tools and supports is an ongoing process for me, and I look to recycle or change up my repertoire at every opportunity.

Meditation. A new one for me. I've only being doing meditation for a while. It took me about four years to be open to trying it, mainly due to the fact that I felt I wasn't in the right frame of mind to take it on.

Like many people, I was of the opinion it wasn't for me, it was for those who are a little out there – and the Buddhist monks, of course. Oh, how I have changed my opinion. Meditation comes in various forms, and many of which I've tried. I felt I wasn't into this whole humming or meditating to music thingamajig (I did try them) but I explored many options before finding the one for me. I tried Kundalini yoga, which I enjoyed but didn't stay with. I tried mindfulness which I found beneficial to a point, but I felt it was too much work. I also tried just sitting with myself and my swirling thoughts but again I wasn't consistent with it. I could see and feel the benefits of meditation, but it was hard. I eventually found the one for me, Transcendental Meditation or TM as it's known. It's simple, can be done anywhere and it's a very important go to tool for me.

Please take note that it's important to remember that whatever you choose to do for your own self-care, it needs to be something which suits you, which you enjoy and which benefits you; we are all very different beings at the end of the day.

Get to know yourself

Do any of us really know ourselves? Are we always doing what is best for us? Hiding behind a mask blocked me from truly getting to know or understanding myself. Funnily enough, I now hope I never stop getting to know myself. I think if I do then I'm predictable, boring, and not really living. Instead, I believe it should be a life-long process. One which is influenced by the passing of time, the environment we find ourselves in and our own wants and needs.

Finding my way back to a place of better mental health took me on a journey of self-discovery, through the good and bad, but ultimately lead me to here; a much better place. I started to feel that I knew myself really well, that there was no more I could possibly learn. I was in a good place mental-health wise; I was getting a handle on it. I was back working, involved in creative arts; acting and writing, being more social, and generally looking after myself. Everything felt comfortable.

And there you have it – comfortable!

You could have the good job, school or college, the happy relationship, the family support, the circle of friends, the gym, the house, the nice car, the list is endless and all feeding into this happiness. There is not much more you could ask for. But have you ever stopped and evaluated your life? If you're happy, then why would you, right? I was of this mindset, feeling that everything was good. Why would I want to pick holes in it and rock the boat? Especially considering where I had dragged myself up from? I was in a good place; my comfort zone.

Let's think about this for a second. If you did stop and evaluate your life, do you think all would as rosy in the garden as you perceive it to be? Would you even, at this stage, be able to recognise when something didn't feel right? Or would you feel as if you were ungrateful if you dug deep into this itching feeling of an unhappiness? You have it all, or so it seems, so, who the hell are you, to be unhappy or unsatisfied?

Or maybe you know you're not truly happy or fulfilled. If so, can you tell what is causing it? Do you set about changing it or do you just carry on through it? Okay, sorry for all the questions but this is the last one I promise, well, for this paragraph, anyway.

Do you, ever just stop, take a step back and evaluate how your life is going? Then if you need to change something, do you change it?

Neil's Notes

Actually, you know what? Pause here for a second and get out that trusty pen of yours and make a list of how you feel, both positive and negative points, in your family situation, relationship, work and whatever else plays an important role in your life.

—◆—

Evaluate your life

In a work setting, we evaluate projects; we evaluate the direction in which the company is going. We, as employees, in turn, are evaluated. Even at school we take exams and they are a guide as to what we need to work on. So why don't we evaluate the direction our life is taking? It makes sense to do this, right? To, check in with ourselves and make sure we are on the path we want to follow. To ensure that we are surrounded by the people we want to have around us.

I wasn't living the life I wanted, which definitely contributed to my mental health problems. On reflection, I think an honest evaluation at certain stages of my life combined with recognising what wasn't working for me, and having a plan on how to change this would have helped me much earlier in my ongoing battles and lack of fulfilment. This evaluation would have allowed me to learn a lot about myself and I do believe I could have made those changes that would allow me to be true to myself and be happier in myself. Of course, it would not have been the whole answer, as I had to consider other contributory factors, but it would have been a massive stride in the right direction.

Thankfully, now I'm open to learning about myself, each and every day. Which means I stop and listen to my mind and body, (yeah, yeah, I know it sounds airy-fairy but it works for me) noticing if my head is filled with heavy thoughts or constant activity which is of no benefit to me. I try to notice if something does not sit right with me; this can be anything that might trigger an episode. If we're honest with ourselves, we know and recognise when something isn't benefiting us. I stop and listen to the signals my mind and body are putting out there. These can be bodily twitches from stress or a heavy head from depression or maybe feeling jittery or it could be sweating from anxiety. There are tell-tale signs I don't ignore.

In hindsight, I do believe my episodes of depression and anxiety, at times, were alerting me to the fact that something or some things were not right in my life. They were reactions to situations in my life which I needed to change, but instead ignored and tried to plough on: Relationships, work, where I resided. It led to me having to make some difficult decisions, but I know they were best for me and in the long-run would benefit me in my life.

What is your depression, anxiety or stress telling you? If you discover this then you can become aware of your triggers and set about avoiding them and or not feeding them.

Some difficult decisions I made involved people. Those who did not add anything to my life but sucked the life out of me. I have distanced myself from some I thought were friends, but realised otherwise. Their friendships drained rather than energised me. I've removed lifelong friends, those I've referred to previously in this book in relation to being excluded from events. Such false friendships. How could a person refer to someone as a close friend, exclude them, time and again, then rub salt in their wounds by recalling the great time they had? These people can do this to me and maybe to you, because they have no respect for me or you, whatsoever.

You get to the stage when enough is enough. When you have to acknowledge the meaning behind those dark times and remove all that feeds them. I've found myself becoming stronger as each day passes, and deciding who I want to have in my life, and what situations I want to be involved in has given me back a sense of control. Now, I will always be upfront about the situation I find myself in: Honest with myself and my feelings, and honest with other people. The beauty of the aging process is that this decision-making becomes a little easier as you give less of a shit about what people think, and come to realise that you don't have to put up with other people's lack of respect for you. As you grow older, you'll realise that you have a handful of true friends. That is what I have now, a handful of good friends, which is more than enough for me. All of whom I've gravitated towards and been open to befriending, because we have many things in common and there is an implicit mutual respect.

Getting to know yourself is about getting to know what's good for you to have in your life, that which offers no benefit whatsoever, and what triggers your times of struggle. It involves listening to yourself. If you worry about pleasing or upsetting others all the time, it will make you sick; simple as.

If you don't agree with something, do you actually know what you should do? Don't bloody AGREE with it. If you don't like something then, again guess what you should do, don't bloody LIKE it. If you don't want to do something, yes you got this, then don't DO it. Do not worry about what others will think. If they care about you then they will respect you, and if they don't, then who cares, they're not for you. When something doesn't make you happy or if it doesn't feel right, then change it or make a decision to move away from it.

Neil, this is easy for you to say now.

It might seem so, but to this day, I still make these decisions, and I know I will do so well into my future. It's not easy to make such decisions but I now know it's necessary in order for me to survive this life and enjoy the beauty that life is meant to bring us. I know I deserve to feel good about myself and not be dragged back down into my dark hole of hopelessness and emptiness by any outside influence.

You deserve all this and more. Don't you?

I was bullied

I am a man, I kept telling myself. I want to believe I'm a strong man. To reveal to you now that I was also bullied, takes a lot. But I've come to realise on this journey that all my reveals and vulnerability is a show of my true strength.

I worked with a few organisations before I decided to work for myself, some being good experiences and some not good. One was particularly awful and consumed my whole being. I was bullied. I should have noticed the warning signs. People before me had left or had been out on sick leave for long periods due to this bullying. This manager wasn't a particularly nice person. Nice in public and to who-ever she felt mattered, but not to us, her *subordinates*.

At first, I questioned whether I was the problem. What could I do better, or how could I be of less provocation to her? It soon became apparent that I wasn't the problem. I spoke to those who had gone before me and discovered that we all had the similar issues with her, and it wreaked havoc with all our lives. She was power-hungry and would micromanage everything, not allowing us leave the office without her approval. If I was doing an email, she would review it and send it back with red lines through the text. Yup, just as if I were in school. She would undermine me in meetings and public settings, which I likened to a parent reprimanding a child in front of his peers. There was no trust; she made each one of us feel like a piece of shit on the sole of her shoe.

A year into the role, and I was being constantly dragged down into a darkness by this person. I enjoyed the work and the interactions with colleagues outside of the office, but over time she eventually wore me down until I could endure it no longer.

I did something I never thought I would, I took action.

I contacted the HR committee and was informed I wasn't the first to do so. While in a meeting with this committee and in full flow putting forward my side of the story, I was interrupted by one committee member. He proceeded to tell me verbatim, 'Well if you were two guys, you would just punch the heads off of each other and that would be it.'

I sat there, stunned. It was obvious nothing would be done on their part. That, in itself was irritating, but what made it even more frustrating was the fact that other people not working directly in the office knew what she was like, having worked on projects with her, but still her reign of dread continued.

I knew I could not continue in this role. I noticed myself being consumed by this, talking about my work situation all the time. When I drove to work, on seeing her car in the carpark, my head would droop, and I would sit in my car for a few minutes to gather myself before going into the office.

I decided to leave. I had no job to go to. I had a mortgage. But I weighed up all of these responsibilities against the impact her bullying was having on my life as a whole and my responsibility to myself. I left. The relief was palpable. It was one of the best decisions I ever made, for me. I put my long-term health first, even when faced with a now uncertain future. I will always make the best decisions for me, for my health and for my life. Will you?

Chapter 17
Lessons learned

I feel lucky to have grown up in Killarney, in Co. Kerry, a beautiful outdoor heaven in the South West of Ireland. Living in a small estate filled with kids of the same age, surrounded by fields, trees and open spaces, which kept us active and engaged each day. I liken our childhood to that of the TV show, the Famous Five (we even had a Timmy, but he wasn't a dog). I have beautiful memories filled with adventure and creativity. I smile and feel a warm sensation when I recall how we would adapt our resources to meet our needs. World Cup year or, well, all year around, we built a wooden goal frame. Wimbledon time, no need for a fancy tennis court, but 'borrow' some yarn from Bridie's treasure trove of wool, tie it across the road in our estate, securing it to the fences on houses opposite. Voilà! Wimbledon eat your heart out. Only one small issue: Games were frequently interrupted by passing cars or families. It seemed like there were no problems for our activities just solutions. This is a mindset I've thankfully reacquainted myself with.

These memories are very much a part of me. And ones that I've carried through all the stages of my life, even if at times they lay dormant and were misplaced. I know they will remain with me well into old age and beyond. We all have them. They might be locked away but they're waiting for you to access them and reintroduce them to your life. The past can bring you some calm in uncertain times. I'm sure if you put this book down, you'll be able to recall some similar childhood memories.

Neil's Notes

Go on, put the book down for a minute or two. Close your eyes and have a wander down memory lane. Don't worry I'll wait for ya! Well, how d'you get on? Some nice memories?

As I introduce you to some of my childhood memories a warm feeling fills me within and makes me smile. The images are now playing like a showreel. I see myself running from our street through our back door and into our kitchen, which is filled with the smell of my mom's fresh baking. She was great. Each week there were fresh scones, brownies, fairy cakes, or madeira cake, to name a few. I would race into the kitchen, starving, in search of a quick snack that I would eat on the run. No way could I sit and eat, as Wimbledon or the World Cup was in full flow right outside of my door, there for the winning. Food in hand, I'd yell, 'Hi Mom! Thanks, bye Mom!' and be gone.

There are so many memories. I remember Sunday calls from my dad. He worked abroad a lot and so Sunday calls with him were like a religion and were, at one time, a source of excitement for the younger me. But, being honest, these became a chore, an unwanted interruption, as they took me away from activities with the lads. One of these calls in particular with him stands out more than the others. It was coming up to Christmas, and we had the same old chit-chat, and then he informed us he would not be home for Christmas. Something every young boy wants to hear, right?

I remember a Saturday in February when I was ten years old, and my father was in our sitting room, packing things into boxes. I stood, confused, outside my bedroom door, my mother in tears; a pain that never left. I watch my father get into his car – my mom crying, tears running uncontrollably down my face – and start to reverse his car out of the driveway; and, in doing so, he reverses over her foot. I see myself looking on as the car moves down the road and continues on out of the estate, me hoping he will notice my tears, and stop. But he never looks back.

I remember wearing a Manchester United jersey at the funeral of a friend, Patrick McSparron. I remember in 1998 having a shower in the changing rooms after a Sunday soccer game and one of my teammates coming in to tell me my friends, Martin Beckett and Sean O'Connor, were killed in a car crash. I remember, in 2005, getting a call early one morning to tell me Kieran 'Cheese' Cahillane had died in a tragic drowning accident in the lakes of Killarney. I remember New Year's Eve 2007, sitting at the bedside of buddy, Johnny Murphy, at Tralee General hospital, making small talk as he nervously waited all day for a promised transfer to Cork University Hospital for a brain scan. He eventually got there, to be told he had an inoperable brain tumour. Johnny died two weeks later, after a rapid decline in his health.

I remember training with Palma Diosi, in Dublin. She introduced me to karate and co-ordination work; I trained her for fitness. I see her never-ending smile and hear her distinctive laugh as I fail miserably at the co-ordination. I remember being told the news that Palma had died.

Even though I remember all of these events and the memories created with these friends and I can feel the pain and the loss they have left behind. Those events hurt like no other pain, but they did not destroy me.

How do I know, you may ask? Well, because I'm here with you, as I write this book. You're reading my words. If they had destroyed me, I would no longer be here. When I delve deeper into what that means, I realise that I'm somewhat resilient. I have experienced pain in my life, but have come through it. I never thought of myself as being resilient but obviously I am.

You might be saying to yourself, alright Neil, jeez, good for you, but I've never had any such pain, or had any real challenges in my life and I feel empty.

My reply to you is simple. You really think you've had no adversity in your life? No challenges to deal with? We all have. They might not be the death of a loved one or some irreversible trauma, but you've experienced something. Some event in my life might have been an incredible struggle for me, but you might not see it as so, and vice versa. So, don't belittle what you've experienced and come through. Acknowledge it, and be proud of the resilience and strength you've garnered from the experience.

Neil's Notes

I can guarantee that you've come through some pain in your life, no matter your age. Have a think, right now. Have you ever had a relationship break-up, have you or someone you know struggled with depression or anxiety or some other form of mental health problem? Has someone you loved died? Have you lost a job or not been successful with a job application? I could go on. I'm sure you've experienced some pain or had some sort of challenge in your life.

So, go on, have a good old rummage in the memory bank, and I believe you'll come up with a few adversities. And guess what? You're here, reading this book. The fact you're dealing with it or coming through it means you've built some resilience, maybe without even knowing it.

—◆—

Control

We will inevitably come up against struggles and face times of great uncertainty as this is the nature of our existence. The COVID-19 pandemic and lockdown is a prime example. If you're still thinking that you're not in any way resilient, well then just have a think about the pandemic and how we've adapted to it. Yes, see, therefore you have become more resilient. Anyway, let's not get bogged down with that, because you'll always be building your resilience. What you do need to do is accept that you'll have challenges. You need to accept the fact that when you're actually in a challenging circumstance and when in it, accepting that it might restrict you and might cause you pain in some way for a certain period of time.

When in this pain, I'm sorry to tell you, you have to accept that you can't control everything. Yes, I said it. You, me, whoever it is, be it the most powerful person in the world, none of us can control everything. Don't believe me?

So, what do we do, do we retreat into our shells and hope it goes away? Do we hide from it hoping it won't affect us? No. We can't afford to do any of that. We need to live and move forward. We need to realise we can still make a choice? Even though we can't control the fact that it's in the world, we can do something that gives us some control. We can choose how we react to the situation. We could recoil and run away, hide and try to wait it out, or we can choose to accept it and adapt our lives which will allow us to keep moving forward. So that means we can always, ALWAYS, no matter the challenge in life, choose how we react to it.

All the events I've mentioned have caused me great pain, and still fill me with sadness to this day. But that's okay. I'm human after all. I do know I've gained strength and built on my resilience from each of the challenges. This will stand to me when the next unforeseen event raises its ugly head. And believe you me, there will be more to come. I'm ready to react, are you?

Chapter 18
Setting a challenge

Of course, as I've shown throughout this book, there are certain situations we can take by the scruff of the neck, and change. What they are depends very much on what blocks or challenges each individual has to cope with. I explored areas in my life I needed to overcome in order to be able to continue to move forward. Even those which were deep-rooted, from childhood.

Some I've overcome. Some are a work in progress, and some I haven't faced yet. Some difficulties that I believe I have addressed successfully still need to be managed. I don't allow myself to become complacent, and let my standards and awareness slip. If I do, it's highly likely that I will fall backwards into my old ways, thoughts and feelings.

The way that I've chosen to face certain struggles is to challenge their physical and mental hold over me. This I do by simply setting challenges for myself. This is a great tool to embrace, because it keeps you focused, drives your motivation, creating a self-learning environment as well as ensuring that you leave your comfort zone, and cross to new unchartered waters. This will allow you to grow as a person. The challenge is set by me, and adapted to meet my need at that time. I set myself up, as best as possible for the win, but push myself beyond my safety net. Each challenge creates more inner strength and confidence and keeps me stepping forward on my new path.

Neil's Notes

What areas of your life are you finding a struggle? Could you set yourself challenges in order to master those struggles? A challenge can be anything you want it to be. I set a no-coffee challenge for a few weeks, which turned into a year and a half, going back to it on my terms. I undertook this challenge to build my staying power and to prove to myself that I'm not reliant on coffee, or anything else, to kickstart my day, that missing my morning coffee won't result in me having an unproductive day. Yes, my coffee challenge taught me all this. Crazy, right! But, hey, it worked for me. Give it a go!

—◆—

Challenging loneliness

I've felt lonely throughout most of my life. Yes, I have a great family and friends, but I still felt as if I was on the outside looking in, quietly suffering and not fully connecting with the people around me. This feeling of isolation was seeded by those traumas already mentioned, and intensified through the wearing of my mask, and the hiding behind the physical walls of my house.

Even though I was now challenging my mental health problems in a more positive way, I knew that many of the contributing factors to those problems – isolating myself, being alone, and feeling lonely – would not evaporate overnight. This will be a life-long process, in which I will have to continuously and actively challenge all contributing factors.

Loneliness, I think, can be both a result and a trigger of depression and other mental health problems. A result, because you deny yourself basic human needs, such as connections and love. I did not let people in; therefore, I never really had this closeness. I did not want to take the chance of people seeing behind my mask. This barrier I had created, in itself triggered a constant feeling of loneliness, even when in company or enjoying activities. This feeling of loneliness was then compounded by my belief that all around me were people enjoying this deep, intimate connection.

This had to change. Failing to do so would mean I was allowing this cycle to continue, and over time it would become more difficult to challenge, eventually dropping me into a well of loneliness that I don't think I would be able to climb out of. As with many of the other contributing factors to my mental health problems, I decided to face this loneliness head-on and challenge it, and that meant I would have to leave my so-called comfort zone behind. In essence, I needed to become more confident and comfortable in my own skin.

As hard as it is to admit, in hindsight I believe I was the creator of much of my loneliness. I often denied myself opportunities to unmask, by saying no rather than yes to invitations and opportunities that would have helped me to override this loneliness.

Weekend dread

I've dreaded weekends for as long as I can remember, having a particular hatred for Sundays. As most people look forward and even live for the weekends, my body and mind would fill with trepidation, knowing that it heightened my feeling of loneliness. This association between Sundays and loneliness stemmed from childhood experience. When I was younger, I often found myself alone on a Sunday. I would invariably be stuck at home to amuse myself as my mother prepared one of her delicious dinners. Sundays were informally known as 'family time', which meant that the kids in my area were gone for the day with their families. I did notice that many of my friends spent this time with their dads at football games or off exploring the Kerry countryside. I didn't have that. No father to take me to the big game or teach me to fish. I dwelled on this as I sat at home, bored and lonely. Don't get me wrong being bored is not a bad thing, it can help you grow as a person, but tell that to 10-year-old Neil. As Sundays came and went and years passed by, I grew to hate Sundays even more.

I'm not sure if you feel the same about Sundays or even the weekend, but it can be such a lonely time of the week for many people.

When in a relationship, I didn't find Sundays as bad, because I had the company I craved, and we often escaped into the countryside. Of course, during this period of time, when in this relationship, it wasn't all plain sailing for me; far from it. I struggled mentally, but somehow, I seem to have blocked that out to some degree, because having company helped me block my problems. When I was single however, I was searching for a relationship for the wrong reasons.

When my long-term relationship ended after 8 years, it created a void in my life. Don't get me wrong, breaking up was the right decision, as we were simply on different paths in life, but we had still shared eight years together as friends, partners, and confidants. We had a bank of memories stored and shared. We had a house together. We were permanent fixtures with each other's families. There was so much that would have to change when we split up. Of course, none of the above should be a sole reason to stay together, but it was only natural to think about all the consequences. I have to admit that after the initial period of relief and excitement, having a weight removed from my shoulders, I didn't know how to deal with it. I began to convince myself that breaking up was the wrong decision, and that, instead, we should get married. How crazy is that? From believing we should break up to now thinking we should get married. I know I'm not the only one who has created such false beliefs. I know of a couple who knew in their heart and soul that they should break up –and they eventually did, thank God, and are both much happier now –but contemplated having another baby instead. Imagine that! It's a tough decision to split, and the easier decision seems to endure and stay together but in the long run it turns ugly. I bought an engagement ring with the plan to propose. It was pure desperation. I was struggling with the new circumstances I found myself in. I couldn't deal with it, because it was a trigger for depression.

I collected my ex from work to go for some lunch and a drive. I pulled the car over to the side of the road. I got out of the car and went around to the passenger side of the car, opened the door, got down on one knee and took out the back box with ring inside. Classy guy, eh! I fumbled my words and tried to explain my love for her and how I believed we should get married and not split. Luckily for me and us, my ex had a good head on her, and knew, deep down, that this wasn't what I wanted. I was so desperate not to face the darkness that lay ahead, I would rather lie to myself and make a mess of both our lives for the next 40 or so years.

So, our long-term relationship came to an end. Thankfully sanity prevailed, but this left me exposed to the darkness ahead. Now, I would not change this decision for the world. This same darkness would have found me if my proposal had been accepted, and we had followed through with a wedding and started a family.

I had lost my first love, the person I had spent nearly every day with for the bones of eight years. Losing the memories, the understanding and that love was hard, and I questioned myself on many occasions. I also had to face my days alone, with this void in my life and, of course, those dreaded Sundays.

Even though I wanted the break up, it contributed to my loneliness and I started to slip into my darkness more frequently. Looking back on it, this was bound to happen, as I was already dealing with mental health problems. My relationship coming to an end, combined with the loss of the escape from reality that the relationship had afforded, and the new reality of facing the void and emptiness became a trigger that sent me on a fast and steady downward spiral into the darkness of depression.

The first week alone was pretty good. I had this freedom (you'd swear I had been locked away for years) and as lads do, I headed out and enjoyed myself. It felt good, going out when I wanted, being able to be somewhat selfish and not having to think about someone else, or watch the clock. I could come and go as I pleased. When in a relationship, sometimes it seemed that the grass was greener on the other side, that I would kill for the chance of a day or two to myself. I had this space now, but that euphoria lasted all of one weekend. I was done with it, I wanted something more, something different, but I wasn't sure what that was. I was lost in the darkness of my depression.

The couch in my sitting room, over time, became my entertainment zone, my dinner zone, my sleeping quarters, my breakfast zone, my nap space and my snack and beer zone. I would find myself couch-bound, not answering calls. There were countless occasions where I would be lost in my duvet on the couch surrounded by pizza, fries, chocolate, coke, beer and, no exaggeration, up to 20 bags of crisps, all different flavours and types. Weekends, particularly Sundays, were back to triggering loneliness and sending me into my deep depression.

The Sunday struggle, I knew, was the first area that needed to be changed. Challenge accepted! My thinking was that if I tried to master being alone on Sundays then it would also have the knock effect of help-ing me get a handle on any other times when I felt lonely. My weekend loneliness was having an adverse knock-on effect on my weekdays, and especially Monday. You know that dreaded Monday feeling? Well, times that by ten, and welcome to my world. I would doze in and out of an anxious sleep all day on the Sunday, not being able to focus on a TV show, picking at the mountain of snacks and drinks stacked around me. Monday morning arrived, and I would be stuck to the couch, trembling with anxiety, faced with the prospect of having to get up and face work. I needed to change this. I needed to confront, once and for all, the hold Sundays had over me.

I needed to figure out how to change my mindset around Sundays. To do this I would need to look back in time, and gain an understand-ing of where this issue with Sundays stemmed from. Okay, we know it's rooted in my childhood. Spending Sunday alone when the rest of the world was, in my head, out having fun and bonding as father and son. But I noticed a pattern from childhood to adulthood. I never tried to change the pattern of loneliness, and move away from it. I would just sit and dwell in it, letting my mind run riot and add layers to it. I never did anything else but dwell, I never took any action or challenged it in any way. Therein lies the answer: Take action. Do something to stop the rot. Be active and stop dwelling. This was what I needed to do. It was time to take action. But what? What action do I take? Not so simple eh! I dwelled in a loneliness I wanted out of, but when push came to shove, I didn't know what I wanted instead.

Alright, focus, Neil. What if I focused on things I like to do? Draw up a list: Go to the movies; enjoy some nice food in a restaurant or maybe just grab a coffee and a cake. List at the ready, all I had to do now was pick one and act on it. The snag was that I had to go and do it alone. How many of us find it difficult to do anything in public on our own? I know for certain I'm not the only. Why go alone you might ask? Well, the reality was that for the foreseeable future I would have to do things alone, as I was single and friends tended to be busy with relationships or families. So, I needed to mirror this reality and, well, do things alone. I also knew I would eventually have to learn how to be able to sit with myself and be comfortable doing so. If I began this process in a public setting it would be less daunting as there would be distractions. I would then, eventually, take the leap to sit with myself at home and learn to be comfortable and even enjoy that.

Decision made. I would go to a pub for something to eat. A pub would allow me to be inconspicuous. I had one in mind that had several entrances and exits, enabling me to slip in and out unnoticed. I arrived at the pub armed with a book. The book was my ally which would occupy my mind and thoughts as I sat alone in the pub.

The idea behind the challenge was to make sure I made choices that would stack the odds in my favour. I had put pressure on myself by believing that if I failed at this challenge, then it would have a detrimental impact on my mental health and my action-taking. Of course, it would affect me but there was more learning here for me, as I had to learn how to pull myself back up from such a set-back. Once I knew the risk and accepted all possible outcomes, then I was ready to face the challenge and all the learning that lay ahead.

Every choice I made for this challenge had a valid reason: A pub with many entrances, so that I could enter unnoticed. I sat near an exit so that I could leave at any time. A book in hand to lose myself in, and occupy my thoughts, but also seem like less of a loser to others in the pub. I arrived and left the pub before the busy lunchtime trade arrived. All calculated moves to favour Neil for the win. I pushed the boat out as I felt more confident. Simple changes on my next visit included leaving the book at home or not sitting near an exit, or going to a pub which was a little livelier. All small changes but for me big, safe steps for my head to acclimatise.

No matter how much I prepared for this, my mind raced and body tensed. I felt as if all eyes were locked on me, loaded with judgment. The menu acted as a shield from prying eyes. As the time passed, I gained the confidence to lift my gaze from my book. I began to focus less on the people around me and more on distractions such as the TV, leading me to more positive thoughts of getting through this challenge. It was already a win! Sure, wasn't I there, eating and sitting alone?

Yes, success, I bloody did it. I won. Bring on next Sunday, I'm ready. Yes, you see this challenge, as yours will be, is a continuous one. Consistency is key when we need to develop a new habit and build on confidence.

Next Sunday arrived. I awoke, opened my eyes, filled with dread as the realisation hit me that I must do it all over again. I did not want to go for pub grub again. My anxiety was through the roof. My mind regurgitated the same old arguments to stop me from progressing. I struggled. It took me an age to get up and get going. I didn't rush myself either but gently convinced myself to move forward.

And off I went. This time to a deli for a coffee and food. I know, not the pub setting but still very much a challenge and, as I always tell people, doing something is better than doing nothing. This was already a win for me considering the struggle I had that morning to get going. I became aware of how I was feeling, knew I had to meet the challenge, so I adapted the challenge to meet my needs that day and ensure a greater chance of success. And that's still a massive win!

As the weeks passed, I began to be less focused on my thoughts, and started to notice other people. Can you guess what I noticed? Yeah, I wasn't the only one on my own. The guy four tables away, he's on his own. Or, that girl there, she's by herself and they seem to be around my age. Ah, the gentleman there, he is at a table for one. Of course, not all those people who sat alone had mental health problems. What they did have in common, as far as I could see, was that they were confident in their own skin.

Give it a try, you won't stand out like a sore thumb if you do things alone. So many people are doing the same.

When is your struggle time?

You might not struggle on Sundays or the weekend. But I'm sure there is some time during the week which you find difficult? Do you find it hard being alone in the evenings or difficult to get up in the mornings? Whenever it is for you isn't the point; what matters is knowing that you can change it by taking action.

You now know that I address this action by accepting the challenge, which inspires me to move. I now do it in all areas of my life. I gave up coffee for over a year by setting myself a challenge; the days I don't want to exercise I set a ten-minute timed challenge; if I feel anxious and can't face work, I again set my timer and challenge myself to do just 25 minutes work.

My advice to you to start small.

It's all about being consistent. Make the challenge weekly and once you feel comfortable at the level you set progress to another level of discomfort. Remember the comfort zone is not your friend, it's someone you meet briefly but leave behind when it's time to move on.

These challenges I set for myself were not easy. They were bloody hard. Each time I felt would be my last; I couldn't go through that experience again. The anxiety and stress the challenge created seemed counter-intuitive, but even if I couldn't see it at the time, they were building my resilience. I could not stop, to do so would halt my progress on my new path. Yes, my new path and these challenges I set were not easy. To this day they, at times, continue to bring me on a roller-coaster of emotions; stress, fear, frustration to name but a few.

However, it did, and does, become easier and some days are easier than others. After the initial apprehension of worrying what people thought, or how it looked when I sat alone, I became more resilient and began to be less concerned. Instead of focusing on those things I could not control (ie, other people), I focused on how I was and how I reacted to these thoughts I constantly conjured up. This was a massive breakthrough for me! Today, my favourite thing to do is go to the movies alone. Get this, I actually prefer going alone than with someone else. I regularly go to eat out alone, I frequently travel alone and explore new places. How times have changed eh! That is the power of consistency and the importance of challenging myself.

Neil's Notes

Let me just state here, these are things *I* like to do. I focused on them because I thought they would be less taxing on me emotionally, and less daunting to undertake as a challenge. What I suggest for you is to find what you like. Those things you feel you could tackle. This should allow for a more favourable challenge with the odds stacked in your favour.

I truly believe, by taking action and doing something, you'll find a better way to live, and the strength to stop letting the worry of being alone, or the fear of being lonely, consume you. We should all be comfortable being in our own company. I'm of the opinion that once you're happy and content in your own skin, then meeting that special someone will be more real, because you'll be entering into a relationship more secure and confident, seeking a true connection rather than just trying to fill a void, or in the hope that this relationship is the missing link to your happiness.

Being alone doesn't have to be forever, I'm at the point now when I enjoy my 'alone' time. Being alone is something we should all try to enjoy. It's a time when you find out more about yourself and what makes you tick. Remember, if you change nothing, nothing changes. You can break the cycle of loneliness and you can break the cycle of being alone.

So, find your own challenge. Be aware that it will be difficult, and work at it. Be consistent and win. Then move onto the next one. I want you to write down some activity that would challenge you, something that will help you grow.

If you find it hard to think of something, answer this question: What is something to which you would definitely say, NOT A HOPE IN HELL am I doing that alone.

Think of a few things and there you have it, your personal challenge!

—◆—

Chapter 19
Taking the new path

I first opened up about my mental health problems in April of 2014. I then took a massive step, eight months later in the December of that year, and began blogging about my journey. I had taken to putting on paper those thoughts that swirled around in my head each day. I noted my observations about my past and present experiences with these thoughts and problems. I felt I was ready and willing to share these writings to the world through my blog.

It would help heal those suffering like I have. It would set them free from their struggles so they won't have wasted years, like yours truly. I was taking a bold step, as once my blog filtered out into the world, I would not be able to hide anymore. No more mask. To make sure this could not be reversed I would name my blog, Neil Kelders. No hiding, just the new Neil saying, 'Hello world this is me. I'm here to rid you of depression, anxiety and those suicidal thoughts forever. Hey, I did it and so can you.'

Yup, I was gonna be the saviour, writing *my* blog for *you*. Before publishing, which I had wanted to do months before December, I discussed it with my family, informing them of my idea and checking to see if they were okay with it, because, remember, this could in a way affect them too. Being given the okay, I was ready to plough ahead, until my oldest brother, Paul, stopped me in my tracks with some interesting questions.

'Why are you doing it and who is it for?'

'No need to think here bro, it's for the world. I will help all those suffering.'

'That's great,' said he, 'but what about you?'

'Me?' I replied, confused.

He continued, 'Do you not think you should be doing it for you?'

After my initial anger and frustration at what felt like him trying to sabotage my great idea, I realised he was right. He was so right. Yes, it's a great thing to do, to share one's experiences in order to help others but I had to be mindful and really make sure if it was right for me at that moment in time. If I'm honest, I wasn't fully ready. When sharing and writing about such experiences, it takes a lot out of a person. It could trigger something, even be a set-back, if I wasn't careful.

Honestly, even writing this book has taken me longer than expected, because I found I had to take extended breaks from the process. It's about me recounting my life while living with deep-rooted mental health problems, and at times that became a little overwhelming.

Slow but steady wins the race.

The times when I felt good within myself, similar to how I felt that day, when I talked for the first time. I wanted to do everything at once. That particular day, I felt I could and wanted to do everything; go running, meet friends, ask a girl out on a date, work on a new project and all at the same time. I wanted to do it all and right now. It was a new feeling and a great one, but not sustainable. I needed to pace myself and that's what I recommend for you.

Take one step at a time. Focus on one thing and take gradual steps with it. Why, you might ask? Well, there will come a period of time down the line when you don't feel as good, and if you've been push-ing yourself multiple steps at a time, then you will, at that moment, feel overwhelmed, which could be detrimental to the progress you've already made. You will doubt your progress and doubt that you can ever sustain such action steps.

As time goes by, you'll experience growth on all levels; self-confidence, resilience, and acceptance of failure to name but a few, but it takes time to build to that level. Don't, as they say, 'put the cart before the horse'. Move forward and progress one step at a time.

My blog

I published my blog when I felt I was in a better frame of mind to share my writings, in December 2014. Oh, do I remember the day! Setting up the blog page, writing up my post, adding pictures, making sure I was nice and ready to release it and share it on my social media platforms. As the day wore on, a panic set in. Trying to convince myself that this wasn't a good idea at all. What was I thinking? I'm not ready to reveal all to the world, to be the topic of conversation to those who know me and I'm not ready to have my name mispronounced by strangers who don't know me from Adam. I'll never be able to take it back; I'll definitely lose people from my life; I'll be the focus of inquisitive eyes; I'm not ready to be judged or felt sorry for; oh, sweet Jesus! This thought-thread continued up until the final moment when, at 2am the next morning, I pressed 'publish'.

Eyes wide open, tossing and turning, I couldn't sleep. I was envisioning people talking about me at dinner, on a night out, on phone calls...EVERYWHERE. In my mind, I was literally the talk of the town. I wasn't ready for this; I didn't want it. Okay that might sound a little strange, I can hear you saying, 'Eh you didn't want it? You released a blog of your own accord, but you didn't want the attention? Ah come on, pull the other one.'

But that's how I felt, and I never said my feelings weren't contradictory! Writing the blog and being open about my mental health issues felt both cathartic and terrifying at the same time, because for 21 years I'd hidden that side of me from the world, not wanting people to notice me. I wanted to share my struggle, and potentially help others, but I didn't want people to talk about me.

Not in my wildest dreams

I eventually fell asleep, mentally drained. When I awoke, I remember my first thought was hoping it was a bad dream. You know, when you wake up, sometimes, not sure if something really happened or not. I checked my social media accounts, yup it was real, alright. FUCK!

Hold on what's this? Messages? Comments on the blog on Facebook, private messages on Facebook, messages on the blog website. Shit, shit, shit! You know it, right, that anxiety that kicks in when you receive an email or text message or any bloody message and you automatically think it's bad news. You sit there refusing to open it.

Eventually I clicked 'open message', then another, and another and another and…. I sat in stunned silence. Not knowing how to react. People I knew were messaging me, 'Well done.' Many wrote that they never would have guessed. More said how brave I was to tell my story. I felt my face reddening, because us Irish can't take a compliment. Some even opened up to me, there and then, about their own personal experiences and thanked me for sharing. All were stunned that I, Neil, this guy they saw as happy, outgoing, active, passionate and funny, was struggling so much and had managed to keep it hidden for so long.

There were messages from people I didn't know, sending someone they didn't know similar heart-warming messages. All of the messages included offers of help and support, *'I'm here if you need to talk'*. That was, well, it was odd and so touching at the same time. I had, literally, just opened up to the world and I found strangers who were ready to support me and listen to me. Over the coming days, as my message gathered legs, more and more people reached out. People can be great; they just need to be given the chance.

Will you give them that chance? I'm glad I did.

I will be honest and say that it did become a little overwhelming. I had to take a little time away from the blog and the messages. Even though they were all positive messages, it became a little too much for me to process. It was mainly due to all this new attention I was receiving. Something I wasn't used to, something not many of us are used to. It's okay to take time out and give yourself some space, but I had to make sure it did not stop me from moving forward. It's important to get back up and start moving again.

The fact that all these people were willing to share and open up to me was truly amazing and inspiring. But I had to be mindful that when connecting with people around mental health matters, I did not make their problems my own, if you get me? This was all new to me, I was still dealing with my journey and might always be. I wanted to help people but I couldn't make their problems mine, this would have been detrimental for me. It would have set me back on my journey.

What struck me about the messages is how many other people also struggled. I'm not alone in this and I don't have to deal with it on my own.

There are people everywhere, people who have even been a part of our lives at some stage, going through what you and I are going through. When you feel alone, that you're the only one struggling; when you feel that nobody will understand, that there is no way out; when you feel you're different to everyone else, know this: You're not! The person sitting next to you right now, the person you share a desk with in work or in school, even the teacher, a teammate, a close friend, your coffee guy – any one of them might be struggling too. You are not alone on this journey and when you open up, you open yourself up to new opportunities, ones you would never have dreamed could be possible for you. Please believe me and see for yourself!

Neil's Notes

So, if you want to help people, my advice to you is that before you get involved, make sure you're comfortable doing so, and that you're mentally in a good place, yourself. This advice goes also for those who don't have mental health issues. The personal information being shared could be quite heavy. You don't want your response to trigger bad experiences and feelings within you. Just be that ear, and listen. Then maybe explore the option of them seeking further help from a professional, or open up to their own family.

—◆—

The stigma is real!

Just to be clear. Not all messages were positive. One message I received which – I can't put this nicely – kicked me in the balls, came via my blog. At this point I was on a high from all the positive messages. The nutcracker message read, *'Go away and kill yourself u stupid cunt.'* This was my introduction to the world of stigma in relation to mental health problems. Being reminded of this message, now, sucker-punches me in the stomach. I mean holy crap, right. I don't think one could misinterpret the meaning behind that message, eh! Out of all messages I received since releasing my blog, which do you think I focused on the most? Which consumed me for days on end, night after night, heck, hour after hour? Well? Yeah, you're right! The negative one.

All my hard work, all the amazing supportive messages were forgotten. The feeling of belonging here in this life was erased. I now began to think all those messages of support were all lies. Those other people also really thought this way and this piece of shit (yup, still makes me angry) of a person was the only one with the balls to say it.

STOP! STOP! I had to stop this rot which was unfolding. It was essential for my future. After a few days of wanting to revert back to the darkness of my bedroom with curtains closed, phone off, smothered under my covers, I had to change. I had to make a choice. Let this PRICK beat me down or keep myself on my new path of living. Oh, just to clarify, this guy or girl remained anonymous. They were not even brave enough to reveal who they were. They hid behind anonymity and the right to believe it's okay to damage someone with words or real hate. I did eventually garner up the strength and belief to stop the domino effect of those words. I made a decision to turn this around, to use it as a major learning for myself, and hopefully for you. I made a video, yeah, another one but this one very different from the first. I wanted to address this. I wanted to show the pain people can cause, even with words.

I wanted to show, first-hand, the reality you might face when you open up about personal problems. Some people won't get it. Some will view you as weak or even want to knock you down. Not everyone will commend you or support you. I realise, today, why people do this. Many of them see something similar in themselves and can't address or don't want to face it, so they prey on those who are brave enough to act.

So how did I get over it? The video was a good start, in order to release my emotions. I then focused on the message itself, and tried putting it into context: It was just one person. ONE! Yet that one person made me question all the others who gave me support. Maybe the positive messages were fake? Again, STOP Neil! By thinking this I'm disrespecting so many well-intentioned people. The second thing I noted, as I was recycling this curve ball of a message over and over in my head, was that we are all entitled to our opinions, every last one of us. And people love to execute this entitlement no matter how misdirected or hurtful to it might be. I can't control what they think about me, but I can control my reaction to it. I need to work on that, and be able to choose to let things go. Things that don't affect me in the long run, and the anonymous person who sent that message, have no more power over me whatsoever. I won that battle!

What deeply saddens me about this action, is that the person who did it has family, friends, colleagues, teammates, any one of whom might have mental health problems, and who might be the recipient of such poison at some stage. The reality is that this anonymous person will be of no help or support to anyone who is suffering. They would not be the individual who'd support someone in their hour of need. They won't be the person who could potentially save the life of that someone they love. That was my reply to the message in the video I posted!

What stigma means, to me

Prior to these personal events, I had often heard this word stigma, and to be honest I truly didn't understand it. What is stigma in the mental health context? Today I'm better placed to answer this, through my first-hand experiences and my work in the area.

I want to share with you one more 'stigma' incident; again, one which caught me by surprise, because it came from a friend. It had been a few months since my big reveal and I was moving one step at a time on this new path.

I had called to this friend one evening for a coffee and a chat. We had not met in a while, as I lived in Dublin and this friend lived back in my home town, Killarney. So, we had not discussed my revelations around my problems. I chatted and my friend listened. After sometime this friend struck up the courage to ask some questions. I'm open to questions because they allow me to keep opening up, and even think about my problems from a perspective I might not have thought about. They allow for conversations to be initiated; they allow for education around the topic of mental health problems; they allow all of us to distance ourselves from the awkwardness and discomfort that inhibits such dialogue. As we chatted, my friend made a statement, which, to be honest, hurt. The friend stated that I was 'attention seeking'.

Attention-seeking

Where do I start with this? First of all, 'dear friend', when I had an episode of depression or anxiety or was feeling low, the last thing I sought was attention. I kept these life-threatening problems under wraps for over 21 years, and you're suggesting that I'm attention seeking? I was stunned!

What really got to me about this statement is that I had known this person for years .They should have known me well enough to know that I'm not an attention seeker .My blood was boiling.

Yes, I can hear you say, 'Hey Neil, listen to your advice yeah? Control your reaction'. Thank you for the reminder (as I give a sarcastic smile).

I could not believe what I had heard. Fair enough, you might expect this from a stranger, but not a friend. Instead of giving me support and trying to understand it further, which can be a tough task, I know – especially as I was a 'smiler' and a joker on the outside – it was dismissed, doubted, twisted. All during our first conversation.

Please be open to listening without being judgmental. It might be hard to understand. So, by all means ask questions and gather the information and facts before you make a decision. I would have more respect for you and maybe I could then understand your statement a little better.

I was pissed off but I did not let it get me down. I heard it, allowed myself to be angered by it, then chose to ignore it. I did take some action to protect myself and the work I had done so far, by distancing myself from this friend. I told you already that I don't need people in my life who doubt me and make me doubt myself, I can do that all on my own, thank you very much! I'm stepping stronger on my new path!

When you start on your journey 'back to your life', you'll have to make such choices. It's not easy but, necessary. Choices about keeping or removing people and circumstances in your life, be it a social setting, at home, in work or any other area where negativity or triggers could infiltrate. You will become stronger, more resilient, when making a decision which has your best interests at heart, whilst also ensuring that you'll have less resistance to deal with as you move along this new path. Remember **YOU ARE WORTH IT!**

Mental health v mental health problems

While on this new path, I've come to realise that I don't need to be afraid of mental health. I'm not afraid of physical health, so why would I be of my mental health? When I have a problem with my physical health, I am concerned, and deal with it. I don't worry about it, otherwise. The same goes with my mental health. When I'm okay, there's nothing to be concerned about.

My understanding prior to this was wrong, plain and simple. When I heard the term 'mental health', I automatically thought: Depression, anxiety, and suicide. So, I hated having mental health. I wanted, so badly, to not have mental health! badly. Yes, go on laugh away, I'll give you that one! Thankfully, I've educated myself on the topic, which was a really important step, as it opened me up to the fact that I could work on my mental health, just as I work on my physical health. I can maintain it when it's in a good state and I can also work on it when there is a problem, again, just as I do with my physical health. That small change in mindset made the world of difference.

This difference struck me during my first visit to my counsellor. I had just opened up to my family about my depression and suicidal thoughts, and an hour later I was on my way to be assessed. As I entered Pieta house, what struck me was how normal everything was. It was a regular day, it was a regular house, with a regular driveway, with regular windows which I could look through. Not what I expected at all. I thought, I dunno, that it would be some like covert operation.

This *is a very serious mental health condition I have, after all. I'll probably have to be brought into the house via an unknown underground car park and gain access to the building through the secret tunnel system, which will lead to a door covered by a big book case. There I will access the room where my undercover sessions will take place. The room will be in darkness until the counsellor enters, because no one can know my identity. This is a MENTAL HEALTH case after all. Heh!*

Well, that isn't quite what happened; you could say I was a little off with my prediction. To this day the normality of that first day amazes me. I was shown a seat in the waiting room, asked if I wanted tea or a coffee. I mean shit, STOP drawing attention to me, do YOU NOT KNOW the gravity of my situation, It's not normal, goddammit. I said this in my head of course. I replied, 'No, I'm okay thanks', and sat there with my brother next to me. A person sat opposite with their support next to them. My head remained lowered so as to hide my face and not make eye contact. Silence filled the room until my name was called aloud by a lady, as she enters the room, reminiscent of being at the local doctor's surgery.

This first visit was eye-opening not only for me but for my brother, too. It opened us up to the fact that mental health was just another part of our make-up as human beings. There was no place for the fictional subterfuge I had imagined.

I began to understand that 'health,' consists of physical health (our body) and mental health (our minds). We have a state of good health, which consists of good physical and mental health, and we have a state of poor health which is made up of poor physical or poor mental health, or both. Health encompasses body and mind, and we have doctors and facilities which cater for both.

I hope this explains a little more about mental health, and the problems that you and I have with it. Accepting you have a problem with your mental health allows you to set about stepping onto your new path. Now you know you can create solutions to the problem and work towards a state of good mental health.

Break time!

At times, I still can't believe how far I've come, and all the changes I've made in my life. I hope my story gives you the optimism to realise that you're worth putting the time and energy into, for yourself. It will greatly benefit the you of now as well as the future you.

As you proceed with the next section of this book, you'll come to learn that having hope is one thing, but benefiting from it in a positive way is another. I hear you ask, 'How do you do this? How do you benefit from it?'

You take action. Use this book as a constant reminder or pick-me-up to do *something*. I don't want this to be a motivational book that gathers dust on your already crowded book shelf, but for it to be your source of action, and as you read, you're actively making choices and changes to your life.

I challenge you! As you read this book, pick something that appealed to you from the pages you've read so far. Then take action to introduce it into your life. Your change starts now! Ever before you've finished reading this book. Are you ready to move on to the next part 'Life'? Let's take a look at how my life is now.

Hey, don't forget the challenge I set you!

See you on the next page!

PART THREE

Life

Chapter 20
I never thought this possible

I need to get this down on paper. My head has that heavy feeling, right now. A tell-tale sign for me that a low mood is incoming. I'm out in a public place but want and need to be hidden away in my home. I don't feel good. But I have tasks that need doing. If I fail to complete them then this will hang over me and eventually attach itself to my low mood and send me into a whirlwind of overwhelm.

I stop, close my eyes, take a breath. Slow down. Breathe. I look at my to-do list and pick two of the easier tasks to complete. I set my timer for twenty-five minutes and work on them. I write, this time in the form of this book. Each and every action I've taken; from stopping, to acknowledging, to writing, are all small wins. They have helped save my day and save me from a sure path of destruction. This is now an automatic response for me.

Once this feeling, which is nowhere near as powerful as it can be, passes, I will reflect. Now is not the time, I'm not in the right place to do so. When I'm feeling better, I will look at what might have triggered this episode. I'm already fairly sure I know; I didn't meditate today or exercise which usually plays on my mind and stirs up a storm.

How cool is this? Me being able to get a handle on a low mood or a bout of anxiety. If I were to tell the Neil of pre-April 2014 that this would be possible, he would have laughed in my face and taken shelter under the darkness of his duvet.

I'm hurt and sad, not jealous

When Shane died in 2013, I experienced a mixed bag of emotions; sadness tinged with a very strange sense of jealousy. It sounds awful to say but I was jealous that he was free from his pain and the uncertainty that the future had in store. Whereas I still had to struggle on and continue to hate myself and life.

Suicide is confusing and difficult to understand, for those who have never experienced the cutting lows of depression. Suicide leaves us with so many questions and the need to have them answered. Why? Why? Why?

In June 2019, I found myself being the one asking the question, 'Why?' On Friday 14th June, I was having an exciting and productive meeting with a production company in relation to a documentary idea I had. I believed it would help so many people. I was walking on air. My voice could reach more people and help them to take action before it's too late.

The next day, Saturday 15th June 2019, I'm brought back to earth with a bang. It's 8.30 am and my phone is ringing. It's my brother, which is strange. I think something is wrong. Mom? His tone is soft. I sense something is up. He doesn't want to come right out and say it, maybe he felt it might trigger something in me.

'Neil, it's –'

Immediately, I knew. He did not have to say anymore. My cousin, Noel Óg (young Noel), as my aunt Róisín would affectionately call him, as we have an uncle Noel, was the youngest of all the cousins on my mom's side. He had taken his life.

I will again reiterate the power of creating memorable moments. They remain with you throughout your life as precious memories. Life moves fast and we don't connect with loved ones as much as we would like. I was lucky, because in the last couple of years the cousins would organise an annual 'cousins' night out'. Always fun, and so natural to be in each other's company. A treasured photo of us all on one of these nights out brings comfort when thoughts are lost.

Noel died aged 35. He had studied and worked in the area of psychology, and was a kind and caring person. He always had a smile on his face and was well able to strike up a conversation in a group setting, something I wish I could do. Easy going and smiling is how he is etched into my memory.

An avid supporter of Bohemians football club and Italian soccer team Lazio, he made many a trip to Rome to cheer on his team. He could also be found on a given weekend cheering the Bohs on from the Jodi stand. Following his passing, in a very touching moment, Noel's name was mentioned over the loudspeaker and a minute's silence was held in his honour, before the next home game. What a beautiful moment for friends and family alike. A cherished memory for sure. Thank you, Bohemians FC.

As with many people struggling with mental health issues, his smile masked his darkness. Noel was more open than most about his mental health problems. One day, a few years back, Noel contacted me to meet up in Dublin City centre. We met in the Starbucks on Grafton Street, across from the famous Bewley's Café. He opened up to me about his depression (I had at this stage revealed mine), and we chatted about our experiences. Like me, he'd studied in university, his chosen course was computer science but, as I had been, he was lost as to what he really wanted to do. He wanted to change career direction and put time into something he had more passion for. He too felt lost at times. We now had more in common than just being cousins.

I often wonder if there had been more I could have done for Noel back then. Should I have been more active, more involved? I regret the fact that I was caught up so much in my own story that I let the connection falter at times, checking in on the odd occasion. I know many people in this situation ask themselves the same question, 'Could I have done more?' It's a hard question to answer, and one not easily put to rest.

My opinion, as I reflect on my own experience with mental health struggles, is that, back in 2014, I didn't believe that anyone could save me. When you're that far gone, all hope is lost. The want for relief and to end this pain is so strong, it's all you truly desire. The thought is constant.

The decision itself, to take your own life, provides a sense of relief. You have made up your mind, with no more indecision. You want more of this relief and believe that you'll only find it in death. Once you've made this decision, probably for the first time in your life, or for a very long time, you feel as if you have control back over your life. You also tell yourself you can't turn back, now. As we know, you can always, without question, at any time, change your decision.

The decision to end one's life is not giving you control back, but if you act on it, sadly, the act can't be undone, hence, all control is lost, forever. I want you to hear that again. When you take your life, it can't be undone. Never! It's an act that the people you leave behind will never get over. Their love for you will last this life and beyond, and so will their pain. I see this pain in the eyes of all of us who have experienced such a loss.

So, another death from suicide has impacted upon me and those I care about. This time the emotions are different. I'm no longer jealous. I'm completely filled with a deep sadness.

The week of Noel's death and funeral triggered me. I fell back into myself, the darkness moved in on me. It made me question if I could truly ever live with my depression and anxiety, or would it eventually get the better of me.

More familiar thoughts of old reoccurred with major self-doubt creeping back. Maybe they have it right. Maybe suicide is the *only* way to be truly free! It's amazing how much control and influence those thoughts can have, even when I had worked hard to distance myself from them for five years.

In 2019 I was in a much stronger place, personally. I was able to and did pull myself out of the darkness and unchain myself from those thoughts. This allowed me to work through the pain and sadness we feel when we lose someone; I was able to mourn the loss of someone special.

I never thought I would say this – but

I don't speak to you from an elevated platform. I'm still at times in the trenches, with you, struggling with depression and anxiety. However, I'm more at ease in my head, more confident in my body, and more present in life. I don't believe I have eliminated depression or anxiety from my life forever, nor do I dwell too much on this thought. But I do expect to be able to manage anything thrown at me, work through it, and move on with my day. I'm much more experienced when it comes to effectively managing my depression and anxiety. I am in the trenches with you, but I know what action to take to help myself. I'm here with you, so use my knowledge and experience to walk with me.

I'm more at peace with myself. I think I've found my place in this life. Oh, and did you notice when mentioning depression and anxiety, not a word did I say about suicide? Now that's progress.

For far too long, I've listened to people on the airwaves, in papers, or books or at conferences speak of beating depression or anxiety. They, like some superhero, have won the war on their mental health problems. It seemed they were now 'cured', hallelujah! But hearing these stories of their incredible transformation did nothing to inspire me. In fact, I felt a disconnect. I could not relate. At that time, I was in my darkness, I was in my struggle but they had, according to themselves broken free, while I couldn't. What a failure I am, right? They were speaking to me from a platform of freedom, something I could not relate to. They lost me. The gap between us was too wide to bridge. My last hope was extinguished as they beamed from their platform. I switched off.

I speak to you from my reality, which is a mixed bag of good and bad, positive and negative emotions, and the highs and lows of my mental health journey. Thankfully, a lot more good days than bad. It might shock you to hear something I never thought I would hear myself say: My depression and anxiety have had a positive effect on my life. Eh! What now?

Yes. Only now do I feel I can make such a statement. I've been through the mill with many a battle. But I have changed my life for the better. My mental health problems were the catalyst for this change. The terrible experiences depression and anxiety have thrown at me have influenced the path I now find myself on. Without them I would never have changed my circumstances.

I now work as a speaker, consultant and coach in the area of mental health and wellbeing, having worked with companies, governments, and on an international stage with the likes of the World Health Organisation. I've written articles for newspapers, and shared my journey on radio shows. So, my darkest moments have now become my brightest light, my struggles have become my passion and career. How cool is that?

The journey with my mental health problems has introduced me to a whole new world. I've started acting and writing. I've met people with a similar mindset, some on a similar journey. These connections highlighted the fact that I'm not as different as I thought I was, to you or anyone else. I just had to, if you like, find my tribe.

Don't get me wrong, it has been hard work to get here, and a continuing task, but I can finally say I'm looking forward to the challenge of living true to myself.

I never thought I would say this, but life excites me, now. To have so many possibilities open to me seems crazy. I know they're there; all I have to do is go get them. I know they're there for you, too. Possibilities are not confined, as we might have thought, to the chosen few. They are whatever you want them to be, discovered on whatever path you choose to follow. Go get them!

Allowing mental health problems to be grounds for not changing is an excuse

You can do this. Believe me, you can! I learned to stop using my mental health problems as an excuse. An excuse not to try to change anything in my life. They dictated the life I was living or not living. My problems allowed me to justify my inaction. Yes, you and I both know how difficult it is to move, never mind spring into action when struggling, but I think you'll enjoy the new lease of life that taking action affords, more so than the current low moods and feeling of failure, right? I know what I prefer and it's not the difficult and restrictive comfort zone of inaction.

Right now, it might be difficult for you to see possibilities other than pain, darkness and constant struggle, but, as I have also shown you, there is more out there for you. You just need to go and get it. Stop hiding behind those mental health problems. Step forward with me.

Once you start, never stop

When you start taking action, don't stop, even when it seems like you're on top of the world. You may well be, so try to keep yourself there, or as close to the top as you can. Maintain your action on every step of your new path.

Maintenance is important, but don't let it restrict you. I learned this the hard way. I had created a comfort zone which allowed me to live a somewhat better life than those previous years spent in a safe and risk-free environment. This zone was essential, initially, for my integration back into life.

Skip ahead two years, and this comfort zone was slowly killing me. I felt my depression and anxiety becoming more frequent and lasting longer. I couldn't understand it. Why was I feeling this way? I wasn't being risky, so why was I falling back into my darkness? I had my same routine day in, day out, and week in, week out. And there it was. It was the same constant cycle. I felt like a hamster on his wheel going around and around, maintaining the pace of the wheel. At times, like the hamster, I fell off, but was able to climb back onto the wheel. That was it. Nothing extra, nothing to excite me. I was bored with what little life had to offer. I was just living, making enough money for my basic needs. I struggled money wise and connection wise. I knew I had to make changes if I wanted to really live. But that would mean taking a giant risk and breaking free of this comfort zone in which I was trapped, exploring dreams and goals, and putting myself into unfamiliar situations, into the clutches of uncertainty. You and I both know that nothing in life is certain, right?

I had to create the life I wanted, take risks, while managing my mental health and breaking free of this debilitating comfort zone. So, yes, I had to stop using my depression and anxiety as an excuse. You might be thinking, 'Fuck you, Neil, I don't use it as an excuse.' Maybe you don't, but you might, like many of us, use it as an objection or an obstacle to actually living the life you want to live and finding a purpose or meaning which will drive you on.

'Are you doing what you want to do in life, are you content?' If yes, then that's great, I'm right behind you. If not, why not? Is your reply, 'Because my mental health...'? How long do you want your mental health issues to stand in your way? Do you see yourself moving away from your current situation? Explore it, and be honest with yourself. Once you feel that you're managing your problems, then I implore you to begin to dream and find purpose in your life. Once you feel there is no joy in your life, even when you have a handle on your mental health problems, then that's the time to move forward.

Chapter 21
Triggers

When I took the action needed to change my life, I not only had to try to manage my depression and anxiety, but also attempt to rewire my mindset. I needed to buy into and believe that I deserved, and could live, a full life.

When I was able, I had to reflect on some past traumas. This does not mean I had to sit in them, as if I were going through them again, but analyse how and why they affected me.

Today I'm very much aware that a trauma in my childhood was a major trigger that was never dealt with, and followed me into adulthood: My father leaving us. I never wanted to admit this, because if I did, I thought it meant he still had some control over my life. By not addressing it, however, control was taken away from me. It hurt to acknowledge this, but I've come to realise that identifying and exploring such triggers, and opening up to what is actually beneath them, could in itself relieve some of the stresses or problems I was facing.

I eventually came to the informed conclusion that when my father left us, this was a trigger for rejection. Beneath this was a feeling of being not wanted, not good enough, never being good enough. This in turn became a trigger for so many of my problems at an early age. This provided an insight as to why I always felt so different, why I found it so difficult to connect with people.

There are many more triggers out there, some in my past, some in my environment now, some in the people around me and some I have not come across yet. I will find them and address them, so as to help myself. Imagine if I had been able to identify such triggers back then, what would my life have looked like? Maybe I would have been able to break free and live or maybe get a handle on my mental health problems and stop them gaining a stranglehold on my life.

Moving forward my way!

We all seem to move through life in similar ways. School, college, job, family, retirement. This is the way we're told it should be done. Work hard, get the best job.

I've had my eyes opened. There are other ways to live.

My way. Your way.

A definite trigger for me and, I've come to realise, for many of us, is a lack of fulfilment with the path we are currently on. I did school, I loved learning but not that way; I did college, a course I wasn't too interested in; I did college again, enjoying it, but not sure if it was a career I wanted; I worked one job, two jobs, three jobs, none excited me, none I enjoyed. But I kept plodding along, unhappy and unfulfilled.

I was doing as everyone else did, live for Friday and the weekend, or Christmas holidays, or the two-week summer holidays. We should be happy with this, right? Work hard and reap the benefits when you retire. It's really mad, when you think about it. Well, for me it was.

For many, work is life. Not for me, not any more. It's one part of my life, one which allows me to enjoy the other parts all the more. Even when I find myself in the lucky position of now being able to work in an area which I am truly passionate about, I'm aware it's still work and so I must be careful not to allow it rule the day. Action is the name of my game and I'm walking in my own shoes on a path of my own making.

The wrong direction

Do you ever think to yourself, what is this big secret that you're not privy to? You know, the secret that others seem to know, which allows them to easily navigate through life, seemingly uninterrupted by their environment or themselves. They have it all figured out and move seamlessly through it.

What was I not understanding? Was there something I was missing? I couldn't figure it out. I imagined every other human having no worries, no fears, and the more I saw their happy faces, and believed they knew what they wanted from this life and were striving each day towards it, the more confused I became.

How do they do it? Why am I not just like them?

As you can see, I automatically assumed I was the one not getting it, the one who was wrong, if you like. This negative mindset contributed to my putting myself down.

My mind is such a strange place at times.

Why did I notice the happiness of others and attribute it as a negative to myself? Why did I automatically draw a personal negative when watching people have 'normal' everyday lives? Well, it's very simple. Because I didn't want what they wanted, and I thought that was a fault in me. Because, why didn't I want what they wanted?

Maybe it's because I've never really known what direction I wanted to take, or where I see my life ending up. This 'not knowing' can be daunting, frustrating, deflating and confidence-shattering. I felt as if I was being left behind. I wasn't reaching the same markers as my peers: College, job, marriage, kids, promotion (college is the only box I can tick). I'm wasting my life! Whenever I measure myself against the perceived norms of society, I always come up short.

Combined with a feeling of being left behind by the masses, I always felt out of my depth. In primary school, I didn't have the confidence to answer maths problems posed by the teacher. I always doubted myself at sports, and never went into a game of football with confidence. In sports, as in life, this leads to an uphill battle from the get-go.

If you let this mindset filter through in sports, in work or in life then you're always starting on the backfoot, working against yourself and giving yourself a tougher path in which to succeed or even just get through the day.

I always felt like a fraud, knowing I would be 'found out', because I shouldn't be on this team, or in this class – honours Maths? Give over! Law? You're in here studying law? You DO NOT BELONG HERE, you fool. I was always beaten before I started; *beaten by myself.* This can still happen to me at times, especially when I begin something new; be it writing this book, or doing a talk with a new company. This is commonly known as imposter syndrome.

This thought process allowed me to plummet to new lows. Leading me to throw in the towel on many occasions in work, play and life. Even when goals were set, they became redundant. I could make even the most clearly defined goals become clouded with indecision and uncertainty. Will I move in this direction, or maybe that direction? So unsure, no clear future I just continued along in the wrong direction. I did a sports degree, half arsed, then a law degree, again half arsed. I decided to learn Spanish, and stopped, then French, and stopped, I decided to play the guitar, and stopped... The list goes on. So many ideas and goals are set and remain unfinished. The majority of things I stopped; the few I completed were now opened to an interrogation, why hell did I want to do this or that in the first place?

Today, I still sometimes lack the confidence needed to trust my choices and capabilities, when trying to push new projects or develop new ideas. At times I wonder will I ever gain it. Will I ever succeed, or will I be lost in this ever-revolving door, questioning, which is 'my' life?

What I do know is, I'm changing things positively in my life, I'm not stagnant. I'm more progressive and more of an action-taker. I'm constantly unchaining myself from my comfort zone, trying and finding new things to explore and if they turn out to be not for me, that's okay, I find something else. I don't continue on with the activity for the sake of it. So, don't fret if you feel lost or feel like you've chosen the wrong path for yourself. Stop. Find out why you're not happy. Ask how you can change it? Remember simple steps followed by taking action.

Chapter 22
Dream big

I stopped, and began to dream. Do you dream about where you would like to end up in life, or what path you would like to take? I didn't for many, many years, as there was no point. Why would I bother with such a futile exercise and create a false hope knowing it was something I would never attain, and expose myself to sinking deeper into my depression. Oh, yeah coupled with the fact I knew I had no future in this world. Oh, how times have changed. Today I dream big. I'm the master of my dreams. Are you?

Living purposefully

I'm writing this book in Paphos, Cyprus, on my ridiculously big balcony with the sunshine brightening up my day. As I lift my head from the laptop, my eyes fall onto the sea five hundred metres or so in front of me.

I found my path. Not a straight forward path by any means, but one which has brought great learning, failing, more learning, and an overall excitement into my life. The Covid pandemic hit us hard in 2020, and uncertainty overwhelmed us but I believe it also gave us a great education: Nothing in life is certain and you make of this life as you want. It gave me the push I needed to take the next step and explore this beautiful world of ours.

A new location to call home is on my vision board which adorns my bedroom wall. No strides had been made towards this vision, that is until Covid pushed me into taking action. I think I would be classified as a digital nomad. I don't think I'm cool enough to be labelled so, but I live abroad, work online, hopefully stepping towards being a published author.

My vision board is my direction or compass if you like, which can change as I see fit, at any time. It feeds me, on a daily basis, with a purpose and meaning I have now created for my life. It takes me on a journey of decisions which have opened up another world to me: Working online, new friends from all corners of the world, reigniting my passion for mountain running, to name but a few. It includes those things I would like to achieve and experience in my lifetime, and is open to change as I achieve goals and/or pass through the seasons of life.

I see it first thing in the morning. It's a constant reminder as to why I'm doing certain activities today, allowing me to create thoughts and dreams about my future. It has helped guide me from my inner emptiness to a more fulfilled existence. It brings a great joy and excitement into my life, knowing I'm going somewhere. I'm no longer lost and if I ever feel as if I am, I stop and take in the wonders which await me. All I have to do is step towards them.

Being awoken by the warmth of the Cypriot morning sun is one such step. As I acclimatise to the light each morning, I open the sliding doors from my bedroom, which lead to a balcony. I walk in the heat of the sun to the hand rail, to look out to the sea which moves before me. An uncontrollable giggle filters out like that of a child waking up on a Christmas morning. I have found peace, now.

Every now and again I have to shake myself to see if this is real. Have I actually come this far? Am I really breathing in this Mediterranean air? I'm grateful to be here. Not just here in Cyprus, but this new life, being alive today. I know that sounds like some corny bullshit. It's not. I don't say it to distance myself from you. Listen to me, connect with me. I was at rock bottom for most of my life. Every day was a struggle. I wanted to die every day. It pains me to think about it. I do worry now and again that that pain will find me again. I can't let that happen. I won't let that happen.

Let me help you find the strength to do the same.

Neil's Notes

There's a difference between deciding to live, and deciding you want to live. Remember, I told you I went to the counsellor initially for my family and not for me? After some weeks this changed. I became more invested in the process for myself. If you don't want to step forward for you, find someone or something you would step forward for. Once I moved forward and made changes, I then worked on myself, and became invested in living, and actually enjoying living.

— ◆ —

Chapter 23
Where to go from here?

What is next for you? I know my story can fill you with what you might think is motivation. It doesn't. Motivation only comes from taking action, so it comes from within. My book is your crutch, your support, maybe even your guide. It's the resource to give you the hope to keep on taking action.

This action for you right now might be preparing yourself to open up to someone about your struggles. It might be exploring what passions are lying dormant within you and, once found, what purpose or meaning they will unearth. The point is, you can do whatever you like! Yeah, I'm going to shout that out again. You can do whatever you like!! If I can, so can you!

Decision time

I didn't rush making decisions. I explored all the choices open to me. I took time over them, made sure I was mindful to choose something not because I thought it was the right thing to do, but because it was right for me. This meant I had to be open and honest with myself. Having the freedom to choose whatever I wanted was liberating, allowing me to take control of my life. I now can dictate my days, and the choices I make are moving me towards *my* goals. It's important to remember that indecision is a great friend of anxiety. When we are indecisive, or even when we agonise over a decision, we quickly begin to unravel as it triggers anxiety and stress. However, when a decision is made, it relieves us of that unwanted stress and anxiety. Make a decision and whatever it is, be okay with it.

I've made some tough decisions. Cutting back on work meant less money, which could trigger my anxiety. I looked at the decision and weighed up the pros and cons. Pros, especially it being essential for my life, won the day. I lived week to week but did so with contentment, knowing it was supporting my steps to a more sustainable future.

Now I had less work, this could mean more time to ruminate in thought, which is not good. I needed something to replace my work hours. I needed to find a good focus, something that would provide a sense of achievement, be something enjoyable, that I wanted to do, and maybe even meet new people. I found acting. I found writing. I found interesting people to work with. This away-from-work time led me to writing this book. It led me to being paid to act. How incredible is that? You might say, Neil, that's work. And it is, but it's not a job. It's me working my passions, filling my purpose for this stage of my life. Now, you might at times revert back to those same negative, self-doubting, thoughts. It's a deep-rooted thought pattern, so it's going to take time and patience to be able to overcome or manage it!

One time, on my way to an acting class, as I sat on the bus, I felt my anxiety filtering throughout my whole body. Heaviness in my head, heart speed increased. It continued as I stayed on the bus. I was nearly at the course location, just a 5-minute walk away. My symptoms were getting the better of me. I pressed the red stop button and got off a stop ahead of time. I crossed the road and boarded the number fifteen bus home.

You will be challenged as you take the action you need to take, even if like me, you made the choice to do something you love. That is the stranglehold these thoughts have. That is why you need to fight back or to circumvent them. I needed to find ways to stop them sabotaging my enjoyment and my life. After that incident, I made some changes to my inner journey. I began taking a book to read or I also tried focusing on my lines for the script. I put these simple steps in place in order to succeed in attending my class. So, they have a purpose. Some will work out, some won't, keep searching for those which do and you'll continue to succeed. As I discovered, it's time and patience well spent.

Neil's Notes

Have you ever tried to give up something, maybe a habit you perceive as bad, but it just seems too difficult? Yeah? Me too! I have a little suggestion for you. Next time you try to give something up, think about what you're actually giving up. We all have habits, be they good or bad, for many reasons. We enjoy them, we associate them with some sort of relief. Maybe you're of the belief a glass of wine is the only way you can unwind. If you want to give it up, it's important to find something to replace the wine as your way to unwind. It could be an evening stroll in nature, or writing in a journal. The point is, you're still doing something to unwind and not neglecting yourself just because you cut out the wine.

—◆—

Get rid of the negatives

One way I've learned to drive through those negative thoughts is to not stop and think. Pressing the snooze button on my morning alarm puts me at risk of one of these moments. I know from experience that if I press snooze, I won't sleep for an extra 5 or 10 minutes; instead, those thoughts will begin to take hold of me and intrude on my day. So, when the alarm goes off, I hop out of the bed and keep moving, knowing that if I stop then I'm more likely to find it more difficult to proceed with my day as planned.

Acting and the creative arts not only lit up a passion inside me, but taught me some valuable lessons, which became a useful tool on this journey of mine, being transferable into my daily life.

'Yes, and…' is one such lesson.

'Yes, and…' is an essential tool for improvised acting scenes, and I also made it a tool for my life. Improvised scenes on stage are performed without a script, and when the scene is in session each character must be open to whatever is thrown at them. For example, the other improviser/character might say to me/my character. 'I saw a flying elephant on my way to work.' If I were to say, 'Don't be ridiculous, there's no such thing,' the scene has nowhere really to go. The end. However, if I replied, 'Yes, and I saw a two-headed giraffe at a bus stop,' then I've kept the scene going, and also opened up a myriad of possibilities for continuation, such as maybe the animals escaped from a funny-animal farm, or that they escaped from a cartoon playing in the cinema. The scene can go anywhere, not being restricted by me thinking it absurd or thinking that something like that could never happen, ensuring that I'm open to all possibilities and opportunities. It gives the performers great pleasure, as it does the audience.

'Yes and…' allowed me to be open to new experiences, learn about myself and meet new people. Also, the great thing about 'yes and…' is that if I'm not sure about something, the event or activity I said yes to, well, I could stop it whenever I wanted. The important thing is to give things a chance, give yourself a chance by being open to new experiences.

Try something new, and do it for you

I love the piece of advice I will share with you now. You will never regret the things you do, only the things you don't do! Think about it. How true is that?

I'm going to challenge you now. I want you to try it when the next opportunity arises or even better, when you create that next opportunity for yourself. Instead of the usual default 'No,' change to 'Yes, and...' See where it takes you and learn from the experience. You won't regret it!

Improvisation taught me that I might, at times, misjudge what people think of me. When on stage with improv, it can feel to you as if your performance is basic and cringeworthy. It seems as if to perform well, you have to put all your energy and creativity into actively making people laugh. But actually, the best scenes and performances are those which are natural. To the improviser, the performance might seem basic, but to the audience, they offer the most connection and appreciation and laughter. An audience laughs when you least expect it, when you feel basic, they see something else. This is the same in life, people see you very differently from the way you see yourself, and from how you believe they see you. Remember the positive messages I received when I first revealed my mental health issues? Let this be a reminder that the narrative we tell ourselves, about ourselves, and about what others think, is usually very misleading and uninformed.

Chapter 24

Life lessons keep on coming

I had started to put myself back out there on the dating scene. This time I felt I had the confidence to be more honest with myself and the person I met. No connection? No problem, move on.

Take learning from all your experiences in life. I can assure you that I'm still learning, every day; some big lessons and some small. Writing this book has been a source of self-discovery. I've learned a lot about myself on a daily basis during this process. It has been a roller-coaster of emotions, even though I'm in a much better place in my life. I've felt like quitting when anxiety gets the better of me. I've been digging up many dark emotions from my past, and that hasn't been an easy task. I've become stressed and anxious, wondering how it will be received, believing that people will be disappointed at my inarticulate jargon.

Through it all I've continued, even when my editor has run the red marker through my work, my thoughts, my life. Again, I've come through it and learned how to handle myself when faced with such situations. My learning and better understanding of myself and this book process is far from over.

I'm interested to learn how I will react and feel once I have this book finally completed. What I do know is that I will experience certain emotions, both good and bad, and that I'm well equipped to manage them, and will use those experiences to propel me forward and look for another opportunity to move outside my so-called comfort zone.

My life in the last number of years has been filled with new experiences. As far as any of us know we have not done this life thing before. Life is full of new experiences for each and every one of us. Treat life's experiences just as a young child does when experiencing things for the first time: Be inquisitive, and continue to learn all the time through trial and error. Never stop being that child!

Sit with yourself

Things in life were looking up. I was keeping myself busy. Too busy to think. And therein lies my next unexpected lesson. It was great that I was getting out there and being active with my passion and people. I had no evening where I wasn't out and about.

Then came the unforeseen trigger. An acting class was cancelled. It was Wednesday evening. It triggered me. My mood dipped rapidly. I recorded myself and you could hear the low mood in my voice. To note this can be a tell-tale sign that someone is going through a depressive episode. It sounds shallow, fatigued and weak.

I know, I know you're thinking, this reaction is a little over the top for a class cancellation. But you have to realise I had relied heavily on keeping myself busy and my mind occupied. This I believed was the only real answer to my problems. It certainly is a strategy which needs to be implemented but not as a standalone. It has to go hand-in-hand with other strategies. I would not have been able to keep this intensity up; I would have burned out, which would have triggered me.

I now had to learn how to sit with myself, alone. An important lesson and one which you'll have to face when ready. Every strategy I use has been introduced step by step and kept within my limits. I introduced one night a week where I had nothing on. It was an evening to spend at home alone. To embrace the boredom and face the fear of sitting with myself.

I had to learn to be okay with being bored and having no plans. I progressed it to two nights and so on. Today, I am able to enjoy me-time. If I'm meeting people say on a Saturday, then the Sunday I have to myself. In fact, now I need that me-time to recharge and just do nothing; watch Netflix, read a book or try a new recipe or clean the house.

Every problem you encounter can be solved by exploring solutions. Sitting with yourself will be challenging at first but once you consistently push the boundaries and find ways to make it easier, you'll find it very rewarding and energising.

Finding life's sweet spot

Life was certainly going much better for me. I didn't just wait around for my depression or anxiety to hit. I was proactive and happier for it. I was back to working more hours; I was being creative through acting and improv comedy, I had more of a social life, and I looked after my mental health.

Things were nice and comfortable, with each week slowly shaping into a familiar routine. And that was the problem, right there! Even though everything seemed rosy I began to get a sense that something was missing. I couldn't shake this feeling.

This 'being comfortable' was initially for my protection so as not to open myself up to potential triggers. At the beginning of my change this was essential for my development but I soon realised that not taking any risks meant that things were becoming monotonous. I was becoming bored with my days and weeks, and frustrated at the lack of variety my life was offering. Was this it? All life has to offer?

Playing it safe was beginning to eat away at me. Instead of progressing anymore and I was just surviving. I was short on money, which in itself would trigger my anxiety. I had not had a holiday for a few years. I was sick of having to decline invitations to friends' weddings. I could feel myself slipping. I needed to make another decision, and change. It was a difficult decision to make as it felt like I was at massive risk of upsetting the good thing I had going, but deep down I knew it was one I needed to take. I had found a new way to live but I realised I needed to start stepping forward again.

I searched for the possibility of new areas to work in. I didn't want to continue in the fitness industry or pursue the route of becoming a barrister at this time. So, I felt at a loss because I was effectively eliminating my whole nine years of university and study right there. I wanted something else. This was a struggle. I, like so many of us, believe that I had to follow the path I studied in college. I didn't want that anymore.

I wanted something different. I didn't know what I could possibly do. I felt such a waster that I was lost with not knowing what I wanted. I was at this stage at 38-years-old. Most people have forged a great career and moving up the ladder by this time. But I was no wiser than I was at 18 years of age.

At this stage I had begun doing some speaking in collaboration with and sharing my story and journey with various agencies and charities, including See Change, which is Ireland's organisation dedicated to ending mental health stigma, and First Fortnight which is a great charity in Ireland that challenges mental health prejudice through arts and cultural action, so as to create more platforms from which to share experiences, and reach more people.

I enjoyed speaking and was comfortable sharing my story. I loved developing creative ways to share my story, and meet new people who have had similar experiences. I felt relevant. I had a passion for it. Things progressed further, I introduced and shared my story through new platforms; talks, articles for newspapers. I even set a goal. To become a recognised advocate and speaker in relation to mental health. People seemed to connect with my words and thoughts. I grew in self-confidence.

Could this be an opportunity here? Could I develop a business in this area, turning my passion into a career? As they say, if you're able to do that, then you will never work another day in your life. I faltered. I didn't believe I could do such a thing. I began to doubt myself. I believed I couldn't charge a fee for it even though many others were. I knew I worked hard to make sure people got the most out of our interactions. I knew people, through feedback, benefited greatly but I didn't have enough confidence to try.

I dared to dream. A friend asked would I come in and speak to a group. I posted it on social media. Another phone call, and I had my second gig. The rest, as they say, is history.

An excitement that had been missing in life now filled my bones but would, at times, overwhelm me and bring me back to my reality of self-doubt and lack of confidence with a bang, reminding myself to 'stay in my box'. This was another challenge I had to try to address and begin to understand myself even more. I would take some exciting steps forward, telling people of my plans, hearing from them how great I was, then nothing.

I would freeze, and not moving forward meant falling back considerably more steps. This happened with many passions, which I voluntarily wanted to pursue; speaking, acting, ultra-running. I would hit a wall and lose focus. This stepping forward, feeling great, the sliding back was defeating. Every now and again I would read in the paper or see on TV people in my area of work succeeding and being so driven. This created a greater self-doubt, a dawning belief that I wasn't meant to succeed. Does this seem familiar to you? It's a similar pattern of thinking to when I was extremely low. Back then I felt there wasn't anything I could do, only remain stuck.

My talks were going well, as were articles for newspapers but I was still struggling, and just living from week to week. I had begun to question some decisions I had made. Cutting back my work hours to save my life had been worth it, and although it was now causing other issues, I would put my hand on my heart and tell you that I would not change the decision. It was best for me and my mental health. It saved my life, enough said.

I persevered, needing belief and the luck of the Irish.

It came. I was being recognised for my work. By 2018, all my work with charities; talks, articles and projects had given me a platform. I was recommended to represent First Fortnight, a mental health charity, for a trip they were organising to Athens for a European Conference on mental health. This was absolutely amazing. It highlighted to me that my work in the area was being recognised. It gave me the pat on the back I needed. (Luck comes from your hard work as much as being in the right place at the right time). It was important that I recognise what I've achieved, embrace it, feel it, experience it and remember it.

This would inspire me to continue on this journey and give me the belief to succeed.

I've gone on to speak with so many organisations and agencies, government departments, and I have now broken into the international arena; speaking at conferences for The World Health Organisation and The European Institute of Gender Equality. Me! Can you believe it? From being buried by the darkness of my thoughts to using those very thoughts to light the new path which lay before me.

Neil's Notes

Never give up. There are, yes *are*, going to be times when you feel like nothing good is happening to you or that things will never change but please don't give up, keep moving forward and things will happen for you.

—◆—

My relationship with alcohol

My friends and I started drinking at sixteen. I was a great drinker. We frequently would have bets or friendly competitions to see who could outlast who at a drinking session. I could outlast a lot of people. We were into sports, and most sessions (nights out, drinking with the lads) revolved around team sport. Oh, the fun, the laughs, the stories. I grew up in a binge-drinking culture so I never had reason to question my relationship with alcohol. I was just doing the same as everyone else, the norm if you like.

I was back in my home town, Killarney, one weekend and having a few pints with my buddies when a friend of mine, whose bar we were drinking in, stepped out from behind the counter to say hi. We were chatting about this and that and my revelation about my mental health, when she asked me, 'Neil, did you ever think you had a problem with drink?'

I stood there, flabbergasted. What, me? No not all. I'm a good drinker, as in I'm well able to put them away (meaning to easily consume a lot of alcohol). It's funny, because in this pub, on rounds with my friends, I had just ordered another for myself, so I was drinking two pints to their one.

Her comment struck a chord. It made me stop and think. On reflection I'm glad she brought this to my attention. I honestly never thought I had a problem. As I said I was just doing the norm; pints to start the night, and vodka and red bull, Captain Morgan and Coke, JD and coke, and so on, until we would be rat-arsed or bananas or shit-faced or whatever term you use. I was a good drinker and would frequently find myself walking home as the birds were singing on a bright morning, which might mean I'd been drinking for 12 hours straight.

To give you an idea of how good a drinker I was: A weekend in our twenties, a session with the lads was called. Even calling it a session should have informed me that maybe drink was a problem. A 7pm start. I can even remember what I was wearing. A grey long-sleeved tee-shirt with Quicksilver baggy cords (they were stylish, I promise). We hit the pubs, then the late bar, which was usually followed by after-hours (you might call it a lock-in, when you're locked into a pub after closing time) in some pub. We could be there until the early hours of the morning. On this occasion I was in there until the bar served break-fast. The buddies I'd started the night with had all gone home, but not me, because I was the best drinker. I stayed longer and had some pints with one of my friends who happened to be bouncing in the pub that night. He was quite fresh (sober) and I was, well, actually you see this is the thing. Everyone would say to me I looked sober. But to tell you the truth I would hardly remember anything the next day. So that can't have been good right?

Myself and my new drinking buddy, set off on another tour of the town, from pub to pub. I'm now into day two, with no sleep and no break from the drink, the same clothes on for good measure. We drank all day, with other friends joining us later in the day. Day becomes night and, you guessed it, night becomes another pub lock in. I continued drinking and did go to a buddy's house around 5am for a short kip. We then had the bright idea to go for food and a pint. The pints kept coming, the craic (fun) was mighty and we were the life and soul of the party. Everyone loves us, or so we think, and I'm now officially the best drinker in town. Day three, and sober as a judge! Yes, I'm a dope! The session ends in the early hours of day four. I finally have some sense and go home. I sleep and wake, a dose and wake. I'm restless, my mind and body are uneasy. I lock myself away from all contact to battle my darkness alone.

Let's think about that question again. Do I have a problem with drinking? Or is that a problem I have with drink? Do I? Bloody hell, did I what! I did not have a typical or obvious drink problem, as in I would not drink every week, but when I did, shit! The four-day binge wasn't a once-off. When out, I could be life and soul of the party, always laughing, always joking, always masking.

I had to change this, as it was mentally and physically affecting me. No, I did not give up drinking. I do still enjoy a pint of Guinness. However, I made some changes. I stopped drinking top shelf. All shots, be they straight or mixed were no more. This was a big change for me, but one that made a massive difference. On a night out when it got to the shots stage, I refused. I would continue to drink my pints, but as the night went on, I had my fill and would find myself calling a taxi and going home. Pints were then replaced by bottles of beer, which eventually became full bottles that I would leave behind at the bar. Now, on a night out, I'm regularly the first to go home and I'm usually home by midnight. Getting home early means I'm fresh the next day and it's not a day wasted by fatigue and darkness. I'm grateful for this, as the older I get the worse the hangovers will inevitably become. I would be just so damn tired and unable to function.

Now that I have a much better relationship with alcohol, I can go for a pint, have one or two and go home satisfied. I enjoy my pint and the company that goes with it. I don't drink to escape my problems or my reality, which would have inevitably multiplied the next day. Sometimes I will go for a pint alone, and have some me-time, which is a much better and healthier relationship all around.

Do you think I had a problem with how I was drinking? Yeah of course I did. If I'm honest, it seemed to help. It got me out of the house and socialising. It allowed me escape my problems, obviously before sending me right back after a session was done. It allowed me to further mask my problems, because no one would ever think that this outgoing, funny, life-and-soul-of-the-party guy, who hasn't a care in the world, would ever have such deep and dark problems.

Maybe some of this resonates with you? Have you ever looked at your relationship with alcohol or some other substance? Maybe it's something to have a think about?

Chapter 25
Some more ideas for you

I want to share as much as possible with you. You'll notice I'm sharing both those things that worked for me and those which didn't. I explored many ways to help myself and move forward. Yes, this is where that responsibility part comes in. I believe that at the end of the day, the best help you can get is self-help. So, once you've introduced into your life important qualities such as being able to talk openly about your problems, accepting those problems and any of the other external supports you might need, it's then time to help yourself. Are you with me? Okay, super, let's do this!

Be productive every day

I'm a great one for those paralyzingly-long to-do lists. To-do's would more often than not remain incomplete and would trigger anxiety. On days when I was low, I realised that it was unrealistic to expect myself to do all those jobs. I even began to wonder if it was actually possible for me to be productive on low days; whether I should just throw my hat at it and allow myself to be non-productive.

That would not have been a good idea, because it would mean I'd be conceding defeat to my depression. Also, I didn't know how long a single episode would last. Which could mean having to allow myself to be unproductive for several days. Not good; too many days lost.

Instead, I had to learn how to be productive on low days.

I started with the basics: Plan each day. Yes, I know it seems basic enough, but for me it's of vital importance. If I don't know what's coming my way on any day, then I can become overwhelmed and lose the day.

When I first set out on my journey, I only planned one day at a time, as planning a month or a week would have, yes, you've got it, overwhelmed me. I would plan to achieve three things a day. Some days this would be as basic as putting on a washing machine full of clothes, emptying the dishwasher and making my bed. Simple, you might even think stupid tasks, but for me they were three major achievements on that day, given the low state I was in. That was me winning my day. The goal was to keep a consistency with this and slowly build on it each day and week.

Of course, some days were tougher than others, but with practice I was able to create a habit of being productive and cultivate this habit as time passed. I had a plan for each day, and a strategy as to how I would achieve my plan, which was to break my day into 30-minute segments. This is the same structure I use to this day. I adapt my productivity to meet my mood and make sure it allows me to win the day. The main difference today is that I'm now able to plan for a week or a month.

Neil's Notes

Do you know how your tomorrow looks? Well, if not, then sit and write down three things you would like to achieve tomorrow. Plan how you will achieve them. Oh, and don't forget to build in a reward system. When you achieve those three 'to-dos' it's reward time. It's always so important to recognise your personal progress. The type of reward is up to you!

Start now, why wait!

—◆—

Be kind

Are you kind? Kindness, for me, encompasses the qualities of being genuinely friendly, considerate, and sincere, while using your time and resources to help better peoples' lives.

Have a think about a time you were kind. How were you being kind in that situation? Who were you being kind to? Now tell me why you were being kind to that person or in that situation. Were they struggling? Were they a little low? Did something happen to them? Did you just think they needed a little kindness that day?

It's so great that you've been kind to someone, the benefit they would have received from you taking the time and effort to be kind might have been life changing. So, would you agree that we all need to show kindness? I think everyone deserves some kindness in their lives, would you agree?

Are you kind to yourself? Yes, you've read that correctly. I'm serious. If you aren't, then why not? Do you not deserve the same kindness from yourself as you show to others? Are you less deserving of this kindness? Oh, or maybe you don't truly believe in this kindness that you show others, which, I'm sure, isn't the case, so you don't bother with it for yourself? Is it stupid and useless to be kind to others, is that it? No? Oh, then I'm confused as to why you don't show this same kindness to yourself. You said it's real, you've said you're not less deserving, so why, tell me why you don't show yourself this same kindness? I didn't think I deserved it. I was very hard on myself. I never gave myself a break. I would put myself down time and again for the smallest of things.

Oh, and don't worry, I get why you might think it strange to be kind to yourself. We believe kindness is only something you show to others. It does seem an odd thing to do, to show ourselves kindness. But I've learned it's very necessary. It's something I needed to learn, and urge you to also to learn it, because if you're hard on yourself then you're potentially blocking yourself from moving forward through your mental health problems. You're getting in our own way. You'll become frustrated and maybe even lose hope and stop believing that you can create change for yourself. You need to be kind to yourself, give yourself a break, and back yourself all the time.

Being kind to yourself can also mean that you accept praise from others, something I still find quite difficult at times. Maybe it's because I'm Irish? We Irish (not all of course) find it difficult to accept praise.

It's very much okay to accept praise and by doing so, it could elevate you to another level on your journey. It could even kick-start your journey.

Am I blowing my own trumpet?

I've not written this book to be the hero of my own story. It's not about me being so close to ending my life to turning it all around. Am I winning at life? Well, first of all, winning at life is a subjective idea. For me this is finding joy in being alive and not having the fear or dread as I drag myself from one day to the next. Therefore, some days, yes, I need to work hard to bring myself through it? But you know what? I want it, I want to dig deep and drag myself through it when need be. I'm up for the fight when times ask for it.

I'm not preaching from on high. I'm not the person who has overcome depression against all the odds. I won't tell you that once you've read this book, you'll overcome your mental health problems. I'm telling you that you can change your current situation and have a much better life.

If someone suggests they can help you overcome your mental health problems and banish them for good, then I say to you be very wary. How can they be so sure? How do they know that you won't experience some triggering events in the future? They can't. What this book will do is give you hope and ideas on how to make the changes for you. But as we know hope without action is not effective. You need to take action. If you accept you as you are and take action, then you, too, can start living again. Don't let this book, and my story, be one which fills you with a fleeting, short-term inspiration.

I'm Neil. A son, a brother, a really, really cool uncle (well I was, until they became teenagers). I'm the guy who found out that his life was worth something and that I owed it to myself to fight back, and to not give in to suicide. I'm the guy who has stopped asking irrelevant questions, like 'Why me?' and 'When will it stop?' and started working on his mental health. I'm the guy who has built a life and continues to do so with or without depression and anxiety, it doesn't matter. I keep moving forward. I'm no different to you.

I appreciate you taking the time to read my story. My story, '*My journey with mental health*', is one that, even when you put this book down, is continuing on a daily basis, with all the highs and lows life brings. But now my story and the challenges I face are less in frequency and depth, and a lot more manageable. I want to be here in this world. I want to be here with you and all the people who matter in life. I want to create so many more magical memories. I want you to have and feel the same.

Motivation does not come first; to become motivated you first need to take action, which leads us to being motivated and then inspired. Grab that feeling and use it to take more action and then more inspiration will follow. This is how I gave hope, substance and meaning to my life, and this is how you can do it, too.

There are many ideas and tips you can take from this book, so don't overwhelm yourself with the idea that you need to integrate them all into your life immediately. Work at your own pace, introducing those ideas which you think might be more relevant or manageable for you, and don't forget that you can adapt them as you need. One change-of-mindset trick that helped me a lot, and that I definitely want you to try is to gain as many wins as you can throughout the day. A win is something you've done that helps move you forward through that day and can have a knock-on effect for your week. I try to live by that rule every day. So, I ensure I have a winning start and a winning end to my day. Can you do the same? Of course, you can. Try it today!

You never know who you will help

I hope you've been able to take something from this book. If it's just one thing, then that's a win. You might read this book and feel that you're not my intended audience but I believe we can all take something from it; as mental health is a part of our make-up and we never know when we might personally encounter some stress, anxiety or maybe even depression. You never know when what you've read in this book might assist or support you or someone you know in a future situation.

You picked up this book to read for a reason, which might become known to you at a later stage. I'm reminded of a message I received from a man living in my home county of Kerry. I'd written an article for a local paper, detailing my experience with mental health problems. His message began by thanking me for my article, and proceeded to tell me how he came to read it. He has a dog who sleeps in a basket in the kitchen. The basket sits atop old newspapers. When it was time to replace the newspaper that the dog had soiled, he noticed the page with my article. In his message, he told me that he really needed to read those words that day as he'd been going through a tough time of late. My words resonated with him and provided the support he needed. This is exactly why I share my message. You don't know how or when your words or story will filter down to those who need to hear them, or to those who need some hope.

I'm now lucky enough, since sharing my story online, to be able to step out from behind my laptop and speak on stages at various events, and witness first-hand how my talks impact on others. I've been kept chatting, gladly, after talks to people who wanted to share a little about their own struggle with mental health problems. People from your typical Irish, country grandmother, a woman you would describe as the rock for many around her, to a girl in her 20's, a mother with more than one child suffering depression, a grieving parent, a mother of a young family, as well as a couple of older adults who should be enjoying their retirement years. It's touching to see and feel people connecting first hand, and to know that I'm not alone in this. We all need this reassurance at times, no matter how far along on your journey we are.

Depression and anxiety, and the destruction they can cause, knows no boundaries. They don't discriminate based on age, gender, or life circumstance. We are not alone in this. You're not alone in this, even though at times, I know, it feels very much the opposite. By accepting and sharing our experiences, we give hope to many people, and help them, too.

You never know who you might be helping when you talk. That very person might be sitting next to you right now, on the sofa, watching TV. It might be your wife or husband, that person who gives you strength each day. It might be one of your children, the very ones who make you smile on a daily basis. It might be a parent, those we owe so much to; it might be a brother or sister. Maybe it's your colleague at work, you know the funny one who makes the work-day that little easier, or your best friend, that person who knows all your secrets and you theirs – or so you thought. It could be anyone, and you might now be able to help them in some way. It's time for you to talk for you and talk for all.

I get by with a little help from my friends

There are many people in our lives who love and support us through thick and thin, something which really became apparent to me when I made my pain known. The fact of the matter is, a lot of the time we don't recognise them for the love and care they have given us and in many situations continue to do so. We tend to take ourselves and people in our lives for granted, especially when younger. Try to change this!

I wouldn't be the man I'm today if it weren't for some important people in my life.

My mom is someone who worked hard to set myself and my brothers up for the best life possible. She gave us all so much and we never wanted for anything. She goes above and beyond the call of a mother and it's something I will be forever thankful for, even if I sometimes don't show it. I've wanted to find ways to repay her for this amazing love and support she gave. One of the ways in which I repaid her was the timing of when I opened up to her about my struggles. She wasn't the first person I opened up to. I felt at my lowest ebb, and didn't fully understand what was happening to me. I didn't want her to be consumed by worry. Instead, I waited until I was in a better place and actually wanted to live life. I waited a few months and having a few good counselling sessions under my belt. Having become a little more confident and open through this work, I felt ready to open up to her face-to-face.

It's something I'm proud of. Some might say it's selfish to keep your mom in the dark for so long. I view it a little differently, as I felt it was the first time in my life that I had some control. You see my relationship with my mom and my brothers was always one where I felt as if I were just the 'baby' of the family. Not their fault, but something I could not shake and move on from. I never truly took the reins to my own life.

We were sitting in a café after a walk. I started the conversation. My mother, to me, has always had an inner strength, which I think became a necessity when having to raise three boys alone. This inner strength shone through once again as I opened up to her about my struggles behind my mask and my new journey to the other side. I felt justified with my decision not to tell her sooner, as I was now able to calmly and coherently answer any of her questions. I was able to show her a new side of me, one with a found strength and maturity.

A second gift I was able to pass to her that day was to leave her knowing that every day I will work on myself and live my best life. Something I think each and every parent wants for their child; for them to be happy and not suffer. My mom is one of my main reasons to keep moving forward.

The other driving forces in my life are my brother, Paul, and his wife, Sinead. These are the people I want to make proud and show them that their love and support has meant the world to me. Sinead and Paul are the parents to my nieces and nephews; Saoirse, Caoimhe, Patrick and Liam, who are a shining light in my life. They have brought great love and enjoyment into our family, and a new way for us to see life. I want to be someone they can look towards for support, as well as being a positive influence on their life journey. As the years have passed, and their own personalities have come to the fore, I'm now being inspired by them and the way they choose to live their lives.

My uncle Noel is one of the kindest people you could meet; always available when someone is in need, when I was in need, for that I thank you.

My aunty Marie, uncle John and cousins Aisling, Brefni and Shane. Thank you for the exciting times I had as a young fella visiting you in Dublin. My aunts' incredible food and being introduced to the stories and lives of my older city living cousins. I have many beautiful memories being in the presence of my older cousins, exciting for a young country boy.

Recalling the beautiful memories I have on visiting my grandparents, Paddy and Mary 'Cis' Daly and my aunty Róisín in Tullamore Co.Offaly. Playing in the big garden guarded from the main road by the tallest evergreen trees my little eyes had seen. Racing into the house, warmed by the fire my grandfather lit each morning at eight o' clock, to gulp the three course dinner prepared by my gran. Thanks for such happy times which kept me safe in adulthood.

My childhood friend, Sean Clifford, even though he now lives in France, has always been there for me. He supported me from day one. Himself, his wife Valerie and daughter Enya have welcomed me into their home, when I needed an escape.

Rob Cronin has been a calming and understanding influence in my life. Myself and Rob became friends some years ago and developed a good relationship. It's funny, because I think, while growing up, both would have said we would never have seen ourselves as friends. We were very different people on the outside.

Many a day Niall Lyne was my company as we drove from Killarney to Tralee for college. A guy with steel determination, has been a friend for many years.

Grainne O' Sullivan kept me sane when I needed it most. Simply by being an ear to listen, or by cooking me a comforting meal.

Kathie Richardson and I met while acting in a short film together and we became good friends. She has kept me active in acting when at times my focus and enthusiasm might have waned.

My fitness business has been an unlikely source of friendships. Will and Jen Townsend, and their daughter, Lucy, have kept me grounded just by our connection each week. Hearing Lucy call me Nene gives me so much joy.

Scott Langley, whose karate studio in Dublin I frequented for a number of years for my personal training, has played a role in my journey. He didn't know me from Adam, but he was very willing to help me out when I needed it most. If he hadn't, I would have had to leave Dublin, which would have impacted my mental health greatly at that time. Thank you Scott your kindness was a turning point in my life and gave me the confidence to keep moving forward.

Palma Regina Diosi, a sensei in Scott's dojo, always had a smile for all who walked through the doors. Her laugh was infectious and could be heard in the next street. Palma took me under her wing and tried her best to introduce me to karate (God help her). Palma sadly passed away on 21st September 2017 and is a huge loss to all who were lucky enough to cross her path.

I'm lucky to have developed great relationships with my clients; in particular, Willie Reardon, Richard Blennerhassett, and Ann O' Connell, who have kept me going over the years, showing a caring interest in my progression, and sharing their vast knowledge and experience through well-grounded advice.

So many more people have had a major impact on my life. The bottom line is: People are good. Given the chance the vast majority will help you, as they did me. We just need to open ourselves up to believing this. We are human after all and connecting with others and offering this kindness and support is what truly brings us joy.

And thank you, dear reader! I know how difficult it might have been to pick this book up and continue to read until the end. Some of my issues and pain might be yours right now, and it's not easy to have someone shine a light on them and bring them to the forefront of your mind. Thank you for having the strength to carry on, and for being open to changing the way you deal with your own issues. Thank you for taking the time to listen to my story, and keep involved until the very end. I know I can go on but, sure, ain't I from Kerry, after all?

Conclusion

Well, you did it! You've made it to the end of the book, an achievement in itself. Now you know my story, no holds barred.

I've been rock bottom and tried unsuccessfully to drag myself through this battered and bruised 21-year journey. I believed there was no hope for me, that I would never change this and experience the other side of life. I thought it was time to go, but I'm still here.

If I'm honest with myself, then I know I did not try everything to help myself or what I did try I didn't give it the consistency it deserved. I let my depression and anxiety win time and again, to the point where I was exhausted and just wanted it all to stop. I felt like I needed rest; I felt like I needed to close my eyes to the world.

As I write this book, I'm in a better place; in my head, in my body, and in myself. I see joy, and have the desire to stay in this world, not to only exist, but to live the life I want. I'm still very much a work in progress. But I deserve to live a full life. And if I do, then you certainly do, too.

Don't let this book be just another sitting on the shelf, gathering dust self-help book. Use the knowledge and experiences I've shared with you to bring yourself back to life. Believe in yourself. Believe that you can help yourself. Believe that there are people around you, some you might not even know yet, who want to help. I think of life as a journey and we all have only ONE ticket. I'm now making the most of my life-ticket.

I don't want to die, I want to live, I want life, and all it has to offer, and I want to live my life my way! The fact that I'm responsible for my own life means that these wants will become a reality, but only if I take action.

I want to thank you for reading this book. You have helped me greatly by allowing me once again to lower my mask. I hope as you read this, it has given you permission to lower yours. Even if just while reading this book. That is a welcome start. Well done you! Remember: If you change nothing, then nothing changes! Do something!

About the Author

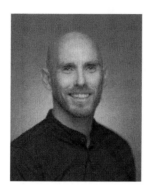

Neil Kelders is a mental health and wellbeing advocate, coach and international speaker, who since his teenage years has suffered from depression, anxiety and suicidal ideation. After 21 years of suffering alone, Neil talked for the first time. Through that simple act, Neil took responsibility through action, and his life was never the same again. His journey has led him to speak to thousands of people worldwide. His mission is to give people a better understanding of what it means to live with mental health problems, and give hope to those struggling to find their way through life.

Contact Neil

Neil Kelders

neil@neilkelders.com

www.neilkelders.com

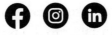

@neilkelders

Leave a Review!

Dear Reader,

Thank you for reading my book. I would love to hear your thoughts on my story and ideas. If you could leave a review on my Amazon page, I would appreciate it, and feel free to reach out to me on LinkedIn, Facebook or Instagram.

If you liked the practical action-steps I included in the Neil's Notes sections, don't forget to download your free eBook, which has additional action-steps and exercises — QR code at the beginning of this book.

Until next time,
Neil Kelders

Made in United States
Orlando, FL
20 December 2022

27362530R00167